Basic Human Neuroanatomy

Basic Human Neuroanatomy

BASIC HUMAN NEUROANATOMY
An Introductory Atlas
Second Edition

CRAIG WATSON, M.D., Ph.D.
Fellow, Department of Neurology, and
Formerly Assistant Professor of Human Anatomy,
University of California, Davis,
School of Medicine, Davis

Foreword by Pierre M. Dreyfus, M.D.
Professor and Chairman, Department of
Neurology, University of California, Davis,
School of Medicine, Davis

LITTLE, BROWN AND COMPANY   BOSTON

Foreword

The study of neuroanatomy has frequently been characterized as esoteric, complex, tedious, confusing, and even irrelevant. Encyclopedic textbooks that fail to separate the minutiae from the core, and poorly organized teaching programs that neglect to present applicable clinical correlations have been in large part responsible for this negative attitude.

Dr. Craig Watson's *Basic Human Neuroanatomy: An Introductory Atlas,* in its revised and expanded second edition, by contrast provides a well-organized, lucid, and relevant introduction to a discipline indispensable to the student interested in the nervous system and the multitude of disorders that affect it.

The impressive illustrations of the intact brain viewed from different directions and the sections of the whole brain, brainstem, and spinal cord at different levels combine with the brief textual account of the organization and function of the nervous system to provide an effective, fundamental exposition of the anatomy of the nervous system. In addition, the illustrations that compare the brain cut in horizontal sections with corresponding levels obtained by computerized axial tomography afford a true and undistorted image of the living brain.

The medical student, the resident training in neurology, and the practicing neurologist will all find that this atlas constitutes a useful and easily comprehensible base for amplifying and expanding their knowledge of neuroanatomy.

Pierre M. Dreyfus, M.D.

Preface

This book was written for one purpose—to be used by students. This may seem obvious, but many neuroanatomy atlases, by their use of complicated stains and exhaustive labeling, seem to be written more for scholars than for students. I made a conscious attempt, both in the text and in the illustrations, to present only the concepts and structures of major importance, suppressing the tendency to add detail for its own sake. It is my hope that this approach will provide a fairly inexpensive but valuable book which students with widely divergent backgrounds and needs (from undergraduates to residents preparing for board examinations) will be able to use in the laboratory as well as at home for self-study.

The book has three parts. The first is a brief review of the organization of the nervous system with a fairly comprehensive presentation of the cranial nerves. I hope that the entire section, but particularly the cranial nerve charts, will facilitate the processes of self-study and review. The second part of the book is a concise summary, in outline form, of the major functional neuroanatomical pathways. Again, it is hoped that this format will enhance the student's efforts to organize the material as well as assist him or her in review. The third part of the book is an atlas of the human brain and spinal cord. The photographs in the atlas are labeled in a way that allows and encourages self-study, self-testing, and review. In order to make the very important correlations between the structure and function of the nervous system, the student is urged to make constant reference to the illustrations in Part III when studying the text in Parts I and II (and vice versa).

Another way of facilitating the study of neuroanatomy is to avoid the use of a stain which reverses the light-dark relationships of freshly cut brain sections. For this reason, the gross brain sections in Part III are stained with the LeMasurier modification of the Mulligan method. This technique leaves the white matter unstained and colors the gray matter blue (dark in a black-and-white photograph). It is a very simple stain to prepare and execute, and a full description of the solutions and technique involved can be found in *Atlas of the Sheep Brain* by R. Glenn Northcutt (Stipes Publishing Company, Champaign, Ill., 1966).

The changes and additions that I have made in this edition are in the general direction of expanding the usefulness of the book, especially for medical students taking their initial neuroanatomy coursework. This will in no way prevent students who want or need less detail from concentrating on those parts of the book that are useful to them, but it will allow those who do want more depth to get what they need without consulting multiple sources.

Aside from minor changes and additions, the major differences in this edition are as follows: (1) the section on eye movements has been rewritten and expanded in light of new information; (2) a series of twelve transverse sections of the brainstem, stained with the Loyez modification of the Weigert method, has been included along with seven new illustrations indicating the position, extent, and relationships of many brainstem structures; also added are (3) a series of eight horizontal sections of the brain cut to correspond, in plane and level, to the standard eight levels of computerized tomography (or CT scanning) of the brain, and (4) a series of normal CT scans to correlate with the eight horizontal brain sections.

The terminology used throughout this book is that which was adopted in 1955 by the International Anatomical Nomenclature Committee and revised in 1960 and 1965. Eponyms are now completely dropped, and the changes agreed upon are generally logical and more informative than the former terms. It is hoped that everyone in the medical community—students, teachers, and clinicians—will now cooperate to make the transition from the old terminology to the new as smooth and rapid as possible.

I thank Robert P. Barber and George Lepp for their excellent photographic work, Celeste Wardin for preparing the illustrations and labeling the photographs, Gerry Sanchez and Ann Wilson for their help in preparing and staining the brain sections, and Linda Royston, whose patience and perseverance in the preparation of the manuscript deserve special gratitude. I am also indebted to Vijaya K. Vijayan, M.D., Ph.D., Department of Human Anatomy, and Nazhiyath Vijayan, M.D., Department of Neurology, for their careful reading of the manuscript, and to Arthur Dublin, M.D., Department of Radiology, for his help in procuring the CT scans—all of the University of California, Davis, School of Medicine. Finally, I wish to thank Mr. Jon Paul Davidson, Ms. Jane Sandiford, and their associates at Little, Brown and Company for their help and support.

C. W.
Davis, California

Contents

I
ORGANIZATION OF THE NERVOUS SYSTEM

The Nervous System

The nervous system is an extremely complex organization of structures that serves as the main regulative and integrative system of the body. It receives stimuli from the individual's internal and external environments, interprets and integrates this information, and selects appropriate responses to it. The parts of the human nervous system that are highly developed (e.g., the cerebral cortex) allow us to use information in a much less stereotyped manner than can the other members of the animal kingdom, thereby presenting the opportunity for humane and cooperative behavior based on rational thought as well as the more automatic survival behavior characteristic of lower animals.

The nervous system can be arbitrarily divided, for the purpose of description, into two large divisions: the *central nervous system* and the *peripheral nervous system*. The central nervous system is composed of the brain and spinal cord, and the peripheral nervous system consists of the end organs, nerves, and ganglia that connect the central nervous system with all other parts of the body. The *autonomic* (or involuntary) *nervous system* is sometimes described as part of the peripheral nervous system, but it really is part of both the central and the peripheral nervous systems. However, to repeat, you should always remember that all these "divisions" are arbitrary and artificial and that the nervous system functions as an entity, not in parts. With that in mind, the organization of the nervous system can be summarized as follows:

Organization of the Nervous System

I. Central Nervous System (CNS)
 A. Brain
 B. Spinal cord
II. Peripheral Nervous System (PNS)
 A. Cranial nerves—12 pairs
 B. Spinal nerves—31 pairs
  1. Cervical—8 pairs
  2. Thoracic—12 pairs
  3. Lumbar—5 pairs
  4. Sacral—5 pairs
  5. Coccygeal—1 pair
III. Autonomic Nervous System (ANS)
 Constituent part of CNS and PNS
 A. Parasympathetic (craniosacral) division
  1. Cranial part—related to cranial nerves III, VII, IX, X
  2. Sacral part—related to sacral cord levels and sacral spinal nerves 2, 3, 4
 B. Sympathetic (thoracolumbar) division
  1. Arises from the spinal cord from T_1 to L_3
  2. Forms the sympathetic trunk with its ganglia

THE CENTRAL NERVOUS SYSTEM

The brain and spinal cord are composed of many millions of nerve cells, or neurons, which are held together and supported by specialized nonconducting cells known collectively as *neuroglia*. Both parts of the central nervous system are composed of two types of tissue, *gray matter* and *white matter*. The gray matter is made up mainly of neuron cell bodies and their closely related processes (mainly dendrites), while the white matter consists of bundles of myelinated nerve fibers (mainly axons). Within the central nervous system, neurons make functional contact with one another by way of *synapses*, whereas they are functionally associated with the structures of the body by means of the peripheral nervous system. The various subdivisions of the embryonic central nervous system and their adult derivatives are shown below.

Divisions of the Central Nervous System

Embryonic Divisions	Adult Derivatives	Cavities
I. Brain		
A. Prosencephalon		
1. Telencephalon	Cerebral hemispheres	Two lateral ventricles
2. Diencephalon	Thalamus, hypothalamus	Third ventricle
B. Mesencephalon	Midbrain	Cerebral aqueduct
C. Rhombencephalon		
1. Metencephalon	Pons, cerebellum }	Fourth Ventricle
2. Myelencephalon	Medulla Oblongata }	
II. Spinal Cord	Spinal cord	Central canal

THE PERIPHERAL NERVOUS SYSTEM

Nervous impulses are conveyed to and from the central nervous system by the various parts of the peripheral nervous system. *Afferent,* or *sensory, nerve fibers* carry impulses arising from the stimulation of sensory end organs (or receptors) toward the central nervous system; *efferent,* or *motor, fibers* carry impulses from the central nervous system to the effector organs (e.g., muscle fibers and glands). Some nerve fibers are associated with the structures of the body wall or the extremities, such as skeletal muscles, skin, bones, and joints. These fibers are called *somatic fibers* and are, of course, both afferent and efferent. Other fibers, also both afferent and efferent, are more closely associated with the internal organs, blood vessels, smooth muscle, and cardiac muscle. These fibers are referred to as *visceral fibers.* As a rule (but not always), most *peripheral nerves* contain all of the previously mentioned fibers (i.e., somatic efferent and somatic afferent, and visceral efferent and visceral afferent), and therefore it is rarely correct to speak of *sensory* or *motor nerves.* It is much more appropriate to use the term *muscular nerve* to describe a nerve supplying a muscle, since, in addition to somatic motor fibers to the muscle, it contains somatic sensory fibers for muscle-tendon sensation (proprioception) as well as visceral afferent and visceral efferent fibers to the blood vessels of the muscle. In a like manner, a nerve supplying the skin should be called a *cutaneous nerve* because it contains visceral efferent and afferent fibers to blood vessels, arrector pili muscles, and sweat glands, as well as somatic sensory fibers for skin sensations. To confuse matters further, some of the structures in the head and neck (e.g., the eye, ear, nose, tongue, and the embryonic branchial arch region) are classically referred to as *special* structures due to the fact that they are not present in the rest of the body. Since these structures are considered special, the structures found in the rest of the body (e.g., regular myotomic skeletal muscle, smooth muscle, glands, skin) are called *general.* So, we end up with *general* and *special, somatic* and *visceral, efferent* and *afferent* fibers in some peripheral nerves. Obviously, since the special fibers supply only head and neck structures, they are present only in (some) cranial nerves. General fibers, on the other hand, are present in both spinal and cranial nerves. All this gibberish falls under the general heading of the "functional components of peripheral nerves" and is summarized below for your reading pleasure.

Functional Components of Peripheral Nerves

A. Cranial and spinal nerves
  1. General somatic afferent (GSA)—Conscious sensation (e.g., pain, temperature, touch, proprioception)
  2. General visceral afferent (GVA)—Visceral sensation (mainly pain; also ischemia, blood pressure, etc.)
  3. General visceral efferent (GVE)—Autonomic motor to smooth and cardiac muscle and glands (parasympathetic and sympathetic; preganglionic and postganglionic)
  4. Somatic efferent (SE)—Voluntary motor to skeletal muscle (derived from myotomes)
B. Cranial nerves only
  5. Special visceral efferent (SVE)—Voluntary motor to skeletal muscle (derived from branchiomeres)
  6. Special visceral afferent (SVA)—Visceral sensations of taste and smell
  7. Special somatic afferent (SSA)—Somatic sensations of vision, hearing, and equilibrium

Functional Components of Cranial Nerves

Nerve	Functional Component	Structure Innervated	Location of Cell Bodies; First Synapse
Olfactory (I)	SVA—smell	Olfactory epithelium in nasal cavity	Nasal epithelium; olfactory bulb
Optic (II)	SSA—vision	Retina (rods and cones) of eye	Ganglion cells of retina; lateral geniculate body of thalamus
Oculomotor (III)	SE	Superior, medial, and inferior rectus, inferior oblique, and levator palpebrae superior Mm.	Oculomotor nucl.
	GVE—parasympathetic	Sphincter pupillae and ciliary Mm.	Accessory oculomotor nucl.; ciliary ganglion
Trochlear (IV)	SE	Superior oblique M.	Trochlear nucl.
Trigeminal (V)	GSA	Skin and mucosae of face and head via ophthalmic, maxillary, and mandibular divisions	Trigeminal ganglion; principal sensory nucl. and nucl. of spinal tract of V
	SVE	Mm. of mastication, tensors tympani and veli palatini, mylohyoid, and anterior digastric Mm.	Motor nucl. of V
	GSA—proprioceptive	Same as for SVE	Mesencephalic nucl. of V
Abducent (VI)	SE	Lateral rectus M.	Abducent nucl.
Facial (VII)	SVE	Facial Mm., stapedius, stylohyoid, and posterior digastric Mm.	Facial nucl.
	GVE—parasympathetic	Lacrimal, sublingual, and submandibular glands; other minor glands and mucosal surfaces	Superior salivatory nucl.; pterygopalatine, submandibular, and diffuse submandibular ganglia
	SVA—taste	Taste buds of anterior two-thirds of tongue	Geniculate ganglion; nucl. of solitary tract
	GVA	Middle ear	Geniculate ganglion; nucl. of solitary tract
	GSA	External ear	Geniculate ganglion; nucl. of spinal tract of V
Vestibulocochlear (VIII)	SSA—hearing	Spiral organ of cochlea	Spiral ganglion; cochlear nuclei
	SSA—equilibrium	Ampullae of semicircular ducts and maculae of saccule and utricle	Vestibular ganglion; vestibular nuclei
Glossopharyngeal (IX)	SVA—taste	Taste buds of posterior third of tongue	Inferior ganglion of IX; nucl. of solitary tract
	GVE—parasympathetic	Parotid gland	Inferior salivatory nucl.; otic ganglion
	GVA	Pharynx (gag reflex), carotid sinus, posterior third of tongue, auditory tube, and middle ear	Inferior ganglion of IX; nucl. of solitary tract
	SVE	Stylopharyngeus M.	Nucleus ambiguus
	GSA	External ear	Superior ganglion of IX; nucl. of spinal tract of V

Functional Components of Cranial Nerves (*Continued*)

Nerve	Functional Component	Structure Innervated	Location of Cell Bodies; First Synapse
Vagus (X)	GVE—parasympathetic	Smooth and cardiac Mm. and glands of thoracic and abdominal organs through transverse colon	Dorsal nucl. of X; many terminal ganglia on, in, or near organs supplied
	GVA	Carotid and aortic bodies; all listed for GVE—parasympathetic	Inferior ganglion of X; nucl. of solitary tract
	SVE	Mm. of soft palate, pharynx, larynx, and esophagus	Nucleus ambiguus
	SVA—taste	Epiglottis	Inferior ganglion of X; nucl. of solitary tract
	GSA	External ear	Superior ganglion of X; nucl. of spinal tract of V
Accessory (XI)	SVE	Mm. of larynx and pharynx (with X)	Nucleus ambiguus (cranial part)
	SVE or SE	Sternocleidomastoid and trapezius Mm.	Accessory nucl. (spinal part) C_1–C_5
Hypoglossal (XII)	SE	Extrinsic and intrinsic Mm. of tongue	Hypoglossal nucl.

Part of Brain Where Each Cranial Nerve Emerges and/or Enters

Nerve	Part of Brain Where Nerve Emerges/Enters
Olfactory (I)	Cerebral hemispheres (rhinencephalon—olfactory bulb)
Optic (II)	Diencephalon (laterally)
Oculomotor (III)	Midbrain (interpeduncular fossa)
Trochlear (IV)	Midbrain (just below inferior colliculi)
Trigeminal (V)	Pons (laterally)
Abducent (VI)	Pons (near midline, just above junction with medulla)
Facial (VII)	Pons—medulla junction (laterally)
Vestibulocochlear (VIII)	Pons—medulla junction (laterally)
Glossopharyngeal (IX)	Medulla (laterally—just posterior to olive)
Vagus (X)	Medulla (laterally—just posterior to olive)
Accessory (XI)	
Cranial part	Medulla (laterally—just posterior to olive)
Spinal part	C_1–C_5 spinal cord (laterally)
Hypoglossal (XII)	Medulla (near midline, between olive and pyramid)

Site of Exit from Cranium of Cranial Nerves

Nerve	Site of Exit from Cranium
Olfactory (I)	Cribriform plate, ethmoid (via olfactory foramina)
Optic (II)	Optic canal, sphenoid
Oculomotor (III)	Superior orbital fissure, sphenoid
Trochlear (IV)	Superior orbital fissure, sphenoid
Trigeminal (V)	
Ophthalmic division	Superior orbital fissure, sphenoid
Maxillary division	Foramen rotundum, sphenoid
Mandibular division	Foramen ovale, sphenoid
Abducent (VI)	Superior orbital fissure, sphenoid
Facial (VII)	Internal acoustic meatus; then: hiatus of facial canal—greater petrosal N.; petrotympanic fissure—chorda tympani N.; stylomastoid foramen—facial N. itself
Vestibulocochlear (VIII)	Internal acoustic meatus (does not leave skull)
Glossopharyngeal (IX)	Jugular foramen (except lesser petrosal N.)
Vagus (X)	Jugular foramen, temporal and occipital
Accessory (XI)	Jugular foramen, temporal and occipital
Hypoglossal (XII)	Hypoglossal canal, occipital

Note: The internal acoustic meatus, the hiatus of the facial canal, the petrotympanic fissure, and the stylomastoid foramen are all part of the temporal bone.

Rapid Neurological Evaluation of Cranial Nerve Function

Nerve	Test	Normal Finding
Olfactory (I)	Apply simple odors (e.g., peppermint, coffee) to one nostril at a time	Correct identification of the odor
Optic (II)	Visual acuity using standard eye chart	Correct identification of letters
	Visual fields using a confrontation test	No visual field defects
	Ophthalmoscopic examination	Normal fundus
Oculomotor (III) (parasympathetic component)	Flash light in one eye at a time	Ipsilateral (direct light reflex) and contralateral (consensual light reflex) pupils constrict
Oculomotor (III), trochlear (IV), and abducent (VI)	Ask person to follow your finger while you move it to the right and left, up and down, and obliquely	Both eyes follow finger in parallel (conjugate deviation)
Trigeminal (V)	Feel the two masseter muscles as person bites down; have person open his/her mouth	Equal contraction of masseters and no deviation of mandible
	Test tactile or pain sensation for all three divisions	Normal sensory perception from entire face
	Jaw jerk and corneal reflexes	
Facial (VII)	Ask person to wrinkle forehead, close eyes, show teeth	Normal execution of the movements
	Apply a small amount of sugar or salt to the anterior two-thirds of the tongue	Correct identification of the substance
Vestibulocochlear (VIII)	Hearing acuity using a watch or a whisper	Normal and bilaterally symmetrical hearing
	Rinne test (tuning fork on mastoid process, etc.)	Air conduction greater than bone conduction
	Weber test (tuning fork on center of forehead)	Heard in both ears equally
	Otoscopic examination	Normal tympanic membrane

Nerve	Test	Normal Finding
Glossopharyngeal (IX)	Touch pharynx with cotton applicator	Gagging (normal gag reflex)
Vagus (X)	Ask person to say "ah"	Both sides of soft palate contract and uvula remains in the midline
	Listen to person talk	Lack of hoarseness
Accessory (XI)	Ask person to turn his/her head to each side and shrug his/her shoulders while you resist the movements	Strong contractions of the sternocleidomastoid and trapezius muscles
Hypoglossal (XII)	Ask person to protrude his/her tongue fully	Tongue protrudes in the midline

The peripheral nervous system consists of (a) the cranial nerves, (b) the spinal nerves, and (c) the peripheral portion of the autonomic nervous system. These three morphological subdivisions are not independent functionally, but combine and communicate with each other to supply both the somatic and the visceral parts of the body with both afferent and efferent fibers.

The Cranial Nerves

The twelve pairs of cranial nerves are attached to the base of the brain (see Figs. 4–8) and pass from the cranial cavity into the face and neck through various openings, or foramina, in the skull. The cranial nerves are presented in chart form on the preceding pages. What these charts do not tell you is where the nerves are located in the body. This you will learn as you study the atlas in Part III, illustrations in other books, and cadaver specimens of gross anatomy and neuroanatomy. In the first chart, the functional components of each of the cranial nerves are listed in the order of their clinical and physiological importance.

The Spinal Nerves

The spinal nerves arise from the spinal cord within the vertebral canal and pass out through the intervertebral foramina. The 31 pairs of spinal nerves are grouped as follows: 8 cervical, 12 thoracic, 5 lumbar, 5 sacral, and 1 coccygeal. The first cervical nerve leaves the vertebral canal by passing between the occipital bone and the atlas; the eighth cervical nerve leaves between the seventh cervical and the first thoracic vertebrae; and the rest of the nerves exit below their respective vertebrae (e.g., the twelfth thoracic nerve exits between the twelfth thoracic and first lumbar vertebrae).

Each spinal nerve is formed by the union of the *dorsal* and *ventral roots* which emerge from each spinal cord segment. It is this joining of the sensory fibers of the dorsal root and the motor fibers of the ventral root which forms the basis for the mixed nature (i.e., containing SE, GSA, GVE, and GVA fibers) of the spinal nerve and its subsequent branches (Fig. 1). Just after the spinal nerve passes through its intervertebral foramen, it ends by dividing into a *dorsal ramus* and a *ventral ramus* (Fig. 1).

Dorsal rami of spinal nerves. The *dorsal rami* of the spinal nerves are smaller than the ventral rami. After they arise from the spinal nerves, they course posteriorly and, with a few exceptions, divide into *medial* and *lateral branches* which segmentally supply the deep back muscles and the skin of the posterior aspect of the head, neck, and trunk.

Ventral rami of spinal nerves. The *ventral rami* of the spinal nerves supply the anterior and lateral parts of the trunk and all parts of the upper and lower limbs (skin and muscles). In the thoracic region they remain independent and segmental in nature, but in the cervical, lumbar, and sacral regions they unite near their origins to form the *cervical, brachial, lumbar,* and *sacral plexuses.* As mentioned previously, the dorsal and ventral rami contain all four of the components of a typical spinal nerve (Fig. 1).

Figure 1. Schematic Cross Section Through the Upper Thoracic Spinal Cord, Illustrating the Main Tracts and Nuclei of the Spinal Cord and the Components of a Typical Spinal Nerve (No GVA Neuron Is Shown)

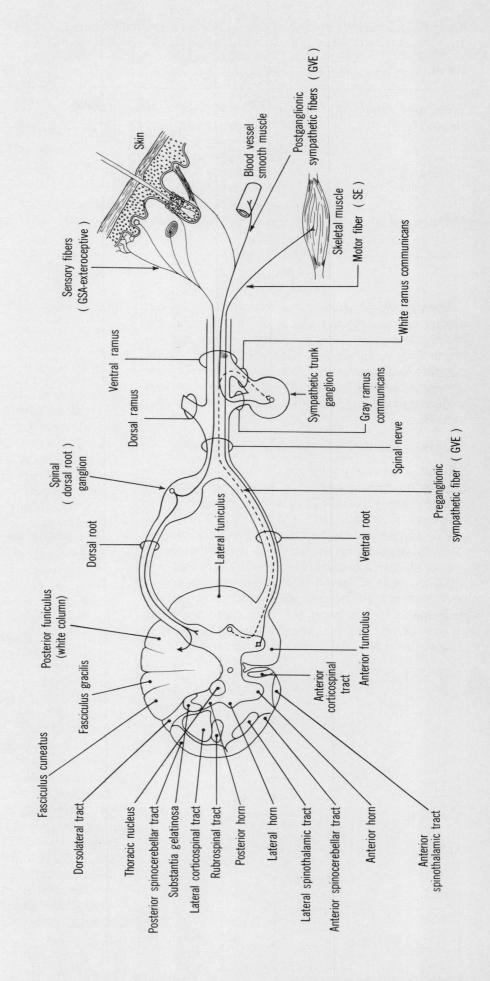

II
FUNCTIONAL NEUROANATOMY OF THE MAJOR SENSORY AND MOTOR PATHWAYS

General Somatic Afferent Pathways

GENERAL SOMATIC AFFERENTS FROM THE BODY

Pain and Temperature

1. Receptors
   The entire question of receptor specificity and the precise matching of sensory modalities with specific receptors is presently unsettled. Therefore, even though I list specific receptors for each modality, do not think that these are the only possibilities or that the receptors given are present uniformly throughout the entire body.
   a. Free nerve endings
   b. End bulbs (Krause and Ruffini)
2. Peripheral processes of unipolar cell bodies (dendrites)
   a. Thinly myelinated fibers in peripheral nerves
   b. Converge on the spinal nerves
   c. Enter the dorsal roots of the spinal nerves
3. Cell bodies of the first-order neurons
   a. Small unipolar cell bodies in the spinal (dorsal root) ganglia
4. Central processes of unipolar cell bodies (axons)
   a. Enter the spinal cord through the lateral division of the dorsal root
   b. Enter the *dorsolateral tract* (Lissauer)
   c. Ascend or descend for a total of one to three segments, sending collaterals into the posterior horn all along the way
5. First synapse (i.e., location of the second-order neuron cell bodies)
   a. Substantia gelatinosa (of the posterior horn)
   b. Posterior horn of the spinal cord
6. Course of axons of the second-order neurons
   a. Cross to the contralateral side of the cord through the white commissure while ascending about one segment
   b. Enter the *lateral spinothalamic tract* (and spinotectal tract) in the anterior part of the lateral funiculus
   c. Ascend in the cord to the medulla
   d. Ascend through the lateral field of the brainstem
   e. At midbrain levels, the lateral spinothalamic tract comes to lie at the posterolateral tip of the medial lemniscus
7. Second synapse (i.e., location of the third-order neuron cell bodies)
   a. Ventral posterolateral nucleus (VPL nucl.) of the thalamus
8. Course of axons of the third-order neurons
   a. Enter the posterior limb of the internal capsule
   b. Pass through the corona radiata
   c. End in the postcentral gyrus (somesthetic cortex) of the parietal lobe of the cerebral cortex —areas 3, 1, 2

Protopathic (Light) Touch

1. Receptors
   a. Free nerve endings
   b. Tactile discs (Merkel)
   c. Peritrichial endings (around hair follicles)
2. Peripheral processes of unipolar cell bodies (dendrites)
   a. Intermediately myelinated fibers in peripheral nerves
   b. Converge on the spinal nerves
   c. Enter the dorsal roots of the spinal nerves
3. Cell bodies of the first-order neurons
   a. Medium-sized unipolar cell bodies in the spinal ganglia
4. Central processes of unipolar cell bodies (axons)
   a. Enter the spinal cord through the medial division of the dorsal root
5. First synapse
   a. Posterior horn of the spinal cord
6. Course of axons of the second-order neurons
   a. Cross to the contralateral side of the cord through the white commissure
   b. A small number of fibers may remain uncrossed
   c. Enter the *anterior spinothalamic tract* in the anterior funiculus
   d. Ascend in the cord to the medulla
   e. Ascend through the lateral field of the brainstem
   f. At pontine levels, the anterior spinothalamic tract comes to lie next to the gracile part of the medial lemniscus
7. Second synapse
   a. VPL nucl. of the thalamus
8. Course of axons of the third-order neurons
   a. Enter the posterior limb of the internal capsule
   b. Pass through the corona radiata
   c. End in the postcentral gyrus (somesthetic cortex) of the parietal lobe of the cerebral cortex —areas 3, 1, 2

Epicritic (Discriminative) Touch and Pressure (Two-Point Tactile Discrimination and Tactile Localization), Conscious Proprioception (Kinesthesis), Vibratory Sense, and Stereognosis

1. Receptors
   a. Meissner's corpuscles—for touch
   b. Peritrichial endings—for touch
   c. Tactile discs (Merkel)—for touch
   d. Free nerve endings—for touch and conscious proprioception
   e. Pacinian corpuscles—for conscious proprioception and pressure
2. Peripheral processes of unipolar cell bodies (dendrites)
   a. Heavily myelinated fibers in peripheral nerves
   b. Converge on the spinal nerves
   c. Enter the dorsal roots of the spinal nerves
3. Cell bodies of the first-order neurons
   a. Large unipolar cell bodies in the spinal ganglia
4. Central processes of unipolar cell bodies (axons)
   a. Enter the spinal cord through the medial division of the dorsal root
   b. Enter the *fasciculus gracilis* (if below the T_6 level of the cord) or the *fasciculus cuneatus* (if above the T_6 level of the cord) in the posterior funiculus ipsilaterally (i.e., without crossing the midline)
   c. Ascend in the posterior funiculus to the medulla
5. First synapse
   a. Nucleus gracilis of the medulla—for fibers entering the cord below T_6 and ascending in the fasciculus gracilis
   b. Nucleus cuneatus of the medulla—for fibers entering the cord above T_6 and ascending in the fasciculus cuneatus
6. Course of axons of the second-order neurons
   a. Form the *internal arcuate fibers*
   b. Cross to the contralateral side of the medulla in the lemniscal decussation
   c. Enter the *medial lemniscus,* which is located just posterior to the pyramids of the medulla at this level
      (1) The cuneate part of the medial lemniscus is posterior to the gracile part as the medial lemniscus is formed
   d. Ascend in the brainstem, with the gracile part slowly moving laterally, then posteriorly, so that by the time the medial lemniscus reaches the midbrain, the gracile part is posterolateral to the cuneate part (other tracts have come to lie next to both ends of the lemniscus by this time also)
7. Second synapse
   a. VPL nucl. of the thalamus
8. Course of axons of the third-order neurons
   a. Enter the posterior limb of the internal capsule
   b. End in the postcentral gyrus (somesthetic cortex) of the parietal lobe of the cerebral cortex —areas 3, 1, 2

Unconscious Proprioception (Muscle Tone)—Two Pathways

A. Anterior spinocerebellar tract
   1. Receptors
      a. Neurotendinous organs (Golgi)
   2. Peripheral processes of unipolar cell bodies (dendrites)
      a. Intermediately myelinated fibers (Ib) in peripheral nerves
      b. Converge on the spinal nerves
      c. Enter the dorsal roots of the lumbar and sacral spinal nerves
   3. Cell bodies of the first-order neurons
      a. Medium-sized unipolar cell bodies in the lumbar and sacral spinal ganglia
   4. Central processes of the unipolar cell bodies (axons)
      a. Enter the spinal cord through the medial division of the dorsal root
   5. First synapse
      a. Posterior horn of the lumbar and sacral segments of the spinal cord
   6. Course of axons of the second-order neurons
      a. Cross to the contralateral side of the cord through the white commissure
      b. A small number of fibers may remain uncrossed
      c. Enter the *anterior spinocerebellar tract* in the anterior part of the lateral funiculus
      d. Ascend in the cord to the medulla
      e. Uncrossed fibers enter the ipsilateral side of the cerebellum through the *inferior cerebellar peduncle*
      f. Crossed fibers ascend through the lateral field of the brainstem to upper pontine levels, enter the cerebellum along the superior cerebellar peduncle, and recross within the cerebellum to the original ipsilateral side of the cerebellum
      g. End in the vermis of the cerebellum
B. Posterior spinocerebellar tract
   1. Receptors
      a. Muscle spindles (annulospiral and flowerspray endings)
      b. Neurotendinous organs (Golgi)
   2. Peripheral processes of unipolar cell bodies (dendrites)
      a. Heavily myelinated (Ia) and intermediately myelinated (Ib) fibers in peripheral nerves
      b. Converge on the spinal nerves
      c. Enter the dorsal roots of the spinal nerves
   3. Cell bodies of the first-order neurons
      a. Large and medium-sized unipolar cell bodies in the spinal ganglia

4. Central processes of the unipolar cell bodies (axons)
   a. Enter the spinal cord through the medial division of the dorsal root
   b. Fibers from spinal ganglia below the third lumbar segment of the cord pass into the ipsilateral fasciculus gracilis and ascend to the third lumbar segment of the cord (or slightly above)
   c. Fibers from spinal ganglia above the first thoracic segment of the cord pass into the ipsilateral fasciculus cuneatus and ascend to the medulla
5. First synapse
   a. Thoracic nucleus (nucl. dorsalis, Clarke's nucl.) of the posterior horn of the spinal cord (from T_1 to L_3)—fibers from spinal ganglia below the first thoracic level of the cord synapse in the thoracic nucleus
   b. Accessory cuneate nucleus of the medulla—fibers from spinal ganglia above the first thoracic level of the cord synapse in this nucleus
6. Course of axons of the second-order neurons
   a. From the thoracic nucleus
      (1) Axons swing laterally to enter the *posterior spinocerebellar tract* in the posterior part of the ipsilateral lateral funiculus
      (2) Ascend in the cord to the medulla
      (3) In the medulla, the tract gradually passes posteriorly, peripheral to the spinal tract of the trigeminal nerve, to enter the *inferior cerebellar peduncle*
      (4) Enter the ipsilateral side of the cerebellum through the inferior cerebellar peduncle
      (5) End in the vermis of the cerebellum
   b. From the accessory cuneate nucleus
      (1) Axons swing laterally as the *external arcuate fibers* and enter the *inferior cerebellar peduncle*
      (2) Enter the ipsilateral side of the cerebellum through the inferior cerebellar peduncle
      (3) End in the anterior lobe of the cerebellum (mainly)

GENERAL SOMATIC AFFERENTS FROM THE FACE

Pain, Temperature, and Protopathic (Light) Touch

1. Receptors
   a. Free nerve endings
   b. End bulbs (Krause and Ruffini)
   c. Tactile discs (Merkel)
   d. Peritrichial endings
2. Peripheral processes of unipolar cell bodies (dendrites)
   a. Thinly and intermediately myelinated fibers in the three divisions of the trigeminal nerve (V), the facial nerve (VII), the glossopharyngeal nerve (IX), and the vagus nerve (X)
3. Cell bodies of the first-order neurons
   a. Small and medium-sized unipolar cell bodies in the trigeminal and geniculate ganglia and the superior ganglia of IX and X
4. Central processes of unipolar cell bodies (axons)
   a. Enter the brainstem at the appropriate level for each nerve (i.e., pons or medulla)
   b. Turn inferiorly and enter the *spinal tract of the trigeminal nerve (V)* ipsilaterally
   c. Descend in the tract through the lower pons, medulla, and into the upper segments of the cervical spinal cord (C_2–C_4)
5. First synapse
   a. Mainly in the nucleus of the spinal tract of V, all along its length
   b. Some of the touch fibers probably synapse in the principal sensory nucleus of V also (see "Epicritic [Discriminative] Touch," next section)
6. Course of axons of the second-order neurons
   a. Cross to the contralateral side of the brainstem
   b. Enter the *ventral trigeminal tract,* which lies next to the medial lemniscus
   c. Ascend through the brainstem in this tract in association with the medial lemniscus
7. Second synapse
   a. Ventral posteromedial nucleus (VPM nucl.) of the thalamus
8. Course of axons of the third-order neurons
   a. Enter the posterior limb of the internal capsule
   b. Pass through the corona radiata
   c. End in the "face area" of the postcentral gyrus (somesthetic cortex) of the parietal lobe of the cerebral cortex—areas 3, 1, 2

Epicritic (Discriminative) Touch and Pressure (Two-Point Tactile Discrimination and Tactile Localization)

1. Receptors
   a. Meissner's corpuscles
   b. Peritrichial endings
   c. Tactile discs (Merkel)
   d. Free nerve endings
   e. Pacinian corpuscles
2. Peripheral processes of unipolar cell bodies (dendrites)
   a. Heavily myelinated fibers in the three divisions of the trigeminal nerve (V)
3. Cell bodies of the first-order neurons
   a. Large unipolar cell bodies in the trigeminal ganglion
4. Central processes of unipolar cell bodies (axons)
   a. Enter the pons through the sensory root of the trigeminal nerve (V)
5. First synapse
   a. Principal sensory nucleus of V in the midpons
6. Course of axons of the second-order neurons
   a. Most fibers cross to the contralateral side of the pons
      (1) These fibers come to lie in close association with the medial lemniscus
      (2) They ascend through the brainstem along with the medial lemniscus
   b. A small number of fibers remain uncrossed and enter the *dorsal trigeminal tract*
      (1) This tract ascends through the brainstem
7. Second synapse
   a. VPM nucl. of the thalamus
8. Course of axons of the third-order neurons
   a. Enter the posterior limb of the internal capsule
   b. Pass through the corona radiata
   c. End in the "face area" of the postcentral gyrus (somesthetic cortex) of the parietal lobe of the cerebral cortex—areas 3, 1, 2

Conscious and Unconscious Proprioception

1. Receptors
   a. Free nerve endings (in joint capsules, ligaments, etc.)—conscious proprioception
   b. Pacinian corpuscles—conscious proprioception
   c. Neurotendinous organs—unconscious proprioception
   d. Muscle spindles (annulospiral and flower-spray endings) in muscles of mastication (possibly facial, extraocular, and tongue muscles too)—unconscious proprioception
2. Peripheral processes of unipolar cell bodies (dendrites)
   a. Heavily myelinated fibers in the three divisions of the trigeminal nerve (V) (mainly the mandibular division)
   b. Pass through the trigeminal ganglion without synapsing
   c. Enter the pons through the motor and sensory roots of the trigeminal nerve (V)
   d. Turn upward and enter the *mesencephalic tract of V* on the ipsilateral side
3. Cell bodies of the first-order neurons
   a. Large unipolar cell bodies in the nucleus of the mesencephalic tract of V in the upper pons and midbrain
4. Central processes of unipolar cell bodies (axons)
   a. Pass from the nucleus of the mesencephalic tract of V back into the mesencephalic tract of V ipsilaterally
   b. Descend in the tract
5. First synapse
   a. Principal sensory nucleus of V—fibers concerned with conscious proprioception
   b. Motor nucleus of V in the midpons—for motor reflexes such as the jaw jerk
   c. Probably the facial nucleus and other motor nuclei of cranial nerves as well
   d. Reticular formation
6. Course of axons of the second-order neurons
   a. Fibers from the principal sensory nucleus of V ascend through the brainstem in the *dorsal trigeminal tract*
   b. Fibers from stretch receptors probably pass into the cerebellum
7. Second synapse
   a. VPM nucl. of the thalamus—fibers for conscious proprioception
8. Course of axons of the third-order neurons
   a. Enter the posterior limb of the internal capsule
   b. Pass through the corona radiata
   c. End in the "face area" of the postcentral gyrus (somesthetic cortex) of the parietal lobe of the cerebral cortex—areas 3, 1, 2

Special Visceral Afferent Pathways

Taste

1. Receptors
   a. Neuroepithelial cells of the taste buds located on the fungiform and circumvallate papillae of the tongue and the epiglottis
2. Peripheral processes of unipolar cell bodies (dendrites)
   a. Special visceral afferent components of the facial (VII), glossopharyngeal (IX), and vagus (X) nerves
   b. Run toward the brainstem in their respective nerves
3. Cell bodies of the first-order neurons
   a. Unipolar cell bodies in the geniculate ganglion of VII—receives fibers from the anterior two-thirds of the tongue
   b. Unipolar cell bodies in the inferior ganglion of IX—receives fibers from the posterior third of the tongue (including the circumvallate papillae)
   c. Unipolar cell bodies in the inferior ganglion of X—receives fibers from the epiglottic region of the tongue and the epiglottis
4. Central processes of unipolar cell bodies (axons)
   a. Enter the pons and the medulla through the roots of the facial, glossopharyngeal, and vagus nerves
   b. Enter the *solitary tract* (tractus solitarius)
5. First synapse
   a. Nucleus of the solitary tract at or near the levels of the respective nerves
6. Course of axons of the second-order neurons
   a. Cross to the contralateral side of the brainstem
   b. Enter the *secondary ascending gustatory tract*
   c. In the upper medulla, this tract comes to lie next to the cuneate part of the medial lemniscus
   d. Ascend through the brainstem in association with the medial lemniscus
7. Second synapse
   a. VPM nucl. of the thalamus
8. Course of axons of the third-order neurons
   a. Enter the posterior limb of the internal capsule
   b. Pass through the corona radiata
   c. End in the lowermost part of the postcentral gyrus (parietal operculum) of the cerebral cortex—area 43
      (1) May also end in the parainsular cortex, which is adjacent to area 43

Smell

1. Receptors
   a. Olfactory hairs at the ends of the peripheral processes of the bipolar olfactory cells
2. Peripheral processes of bipolar cell bodies (dendrites)
   a. The peripheral processes of the bipolar olfactory cells
3. Cell bodies of the first-order neurons
   a. The cell bodies of the bipolar olfactory cells located in the olfactory region (or epithelium) of the nasal cavity
4. Central processes of bipolar cell bodies (axons)
   a. Delicate central processes (olfactory fila) of the olfactory cells collect into bundles (collectively known as the olfactory nerve [I])
   b. Pass through the olfactory foramina of the cribriform plate of the ethmoid
   c. Enter the olfactory bulb, which lies on the cribriform plate
5. First synapse
   a. Mitral and tufted cells of the olfactory bulb
6. Course of axons of the second-order neurons
   a. Enter the *olfactory tract*
   b. The olfactory tract divides into the *medial* and *lateral olfactory striae*
   c. Medial olfactory stria
      (1) Fibers entering this tract terminate in the septum pellucidum, the anterior perforated substance, the subcallosal area, the parateriminal gyrus, and the contralateral olfactory bulb
   d. Lateral olfactory stria
      (1) Fibers entering this tract terminate in the prepyriform cortex and in parts of the amygdaloid nucleus (also in small nuclear groups along the way)
7. Second synapse
   a. The prepyriform cortex and the periamygdaloid area (which receive fibers from the lateral olfactory stria) constitute the *primary olfactory cortex*
8. Course of axons of the third-order neurons
   a. Axons of cell bodies located in the prepyriform cortex project to the entorhinal cortex (area 28), which is regarded as the *secondary olfactory cortex*

Note: The prepyriform cortex, the periamygdaloid area, and the entorhinal cortex collectively make up what is known as the *pyriform lobe.* Structurally speaking, the pyriform lobe includes the anterior part of the parahippocampal gyrus, the uncus, and part of the lateral olfactory stria.

It should also be noted that, although I used the three-neuron pattern for descriptive purposes previously, there undoubtedly are many instances of more than two synapses between the receptors and the cortex in the olfactory system.

Special Somatic Afferent Pathways

Vision

1. Receptors
   a. Rods (for black and white vision and vision in the dark) and cones (for color vision and sharp vision) located in the retina of the eyeball
2. Peripheral processes of bipolar cell bodies (dendrites)
   a. The rods and cones have short central processes which synapse with the dendrites of the bipolar cells of the retina
3. Cell bodies of the first-order neurons
   a. Bipolar cells located in the retina
4. Central processes of bipolar cell bodies (axons)
   a. Remain in the retina
5. First synapse
   a. This synapse occurs between the axons of the bipolar cells and the dendrites or cell bodies of the ganglion cells of the retina
6. Course of axons of the second-order neurons
   a. Converge on the optic disc (blind spot) of the eyeball
   b. Leave the eyeball to enter the optic nerve (II)
   c. Leave the orbit through the optic canal of the sphenoid
   d. The two optic nerves come together at the *optic chiasma*
      (1) In the optic chiasma the fibers whose (ganglion) cell bodies are located in the medial half of each eyeball cross to the contralateral side; whereas the fibers from the lateral half of the retina remain uncrossed
   e. After this partial crossing in the chiasma, the fibers enter the *optic tracts,* which course around the lateral sides of the diencephalon and end in the lateral geniculate bodies
7. Second synapse
   a. Lateral geniculate body of the thalamus
8. Course of axons of the third-order neurons
   a. Enter the *geniculocalcarine tract* (or *optic radiations*)
   b. Pass through the retrolenticular part of the internal capsule
   c. End in the visual cortex on the superior and inferior lips of the calcarine sulcus (on the medial side of the occipital lobe and around the occipital pole onto the most posterior aspect of the lateral surface of the occipital lobe)—area 17
   d. Areas 18 and 19, comprising the rest of the medial and lateral surfaces of the occipital lobe, are called the *visual association areas* and must be intact if you are to interpret what you see

Visual (Parasympathetic) Reflexes

A. Pupillary light reflexes
   When a light is shined into one eye, both pupils constrict. The response of the eye into which the light was shined is termed a *direct light reflex,* whereas the response of the contralateral eye is called a *consensual light reflex.* The pathway involved in both of these reflexes utilizes the visual pathway just presented at its onset.
   1. Afferent limb of the reflex
      a. Fibers from the ganglion cells of the stimulated retina enter the optic nerve, optic chiasma, and both optic tracts
      b. Some of these fibers, rather than synapsing in the lateral geniculate body, enter the *brachium of the superior colliculus* and end in the superior collicular and pretectal nuclei of the midbrain
   2. Internuncial neurons
      a. Axons from the pretectal cell bodies
         (1) Communicate with the contralateral pretectal nuclei through the posterior commissure, and
         (2) Course anteriorly in the midbrain to end in the ipsilateral and the contralateral accessory oculomotor nucleus
      b. Note that light shined in one eye has, to this point in the reflex pathway, crossed the midline (at least partially) in three locations (i.e., the optic chiasma, the posterior commissure, and the tract between the pretectal nuclei and the accessory oculomotor nuclei). This crossing is the basis for the consensual light reflex; while the uncrossed fibers at each of these locations form the basis for the direct light reflex.
   3. Efferent limb of the reflex
      a. Axons from the cells of the accessory oculomotor nucleus enter the ipsilateral oculomotor nerve as parasympathetic preganglionics (GVE) and run with the nerve into the orbit
      b. In the orbit these fibers enter the ciliary ganglion (through the oculomotor root of the ciliary ganglion) and synapse with the postganglionic neurons of the ganglion
      c. Axons of these cells run forward (as short ciliary nerves) and pierce the sclera of the eyeball

d. These fibers eventually innervate the smooth muscle fibers of the sphincter pupillae muscle of the iris

B. Accommodation

When a person who is looking at something off in the distance quickly focuses on an object nearby, a complex reaction called *accommodation* occurs. Accommodation consists of three processes: convergence of the eyeballs, constriction of the pupil, and thickening of the lens for near vision.

There are two theories concerning the mechanism of accommodation. One theory is that accommodation follows convergence, being initiated by it; while the other holds that accommodation occurs simultaneously with convergence. The latter theory will be explained here, but the pathways are not too different for the former theory.

1. Afferent limb of the reflex
   a. Light on the retina evokes impulses which travel by way of the regular visual pathways to area 17 of the cortex
   b. Impulses probably also reach the superior colliculus (and pretectal nuclei) through the brachium of the superior colliculus (as in the light reflexes above)
2. Internuncial neurons
   a. From area 17, impulses travel to areas 18 and 19 and, from there, to the superior colliculus
   b. Tectooculomotor fibers travel to the accessory oculomotor nucleus and the oculomotor nucleus
3. Efferent limb of the reflex
   a. Fibers from the cells of the accessory oculomotor nucleus enter the oculomotor nerve (III) as parasympathetic preganglionics (GVE)
      (1) These fibers enter the orbit and synapse in the ciliary ganglion with parasympathetic postganglionic neurons
      (2) Postganglionic fibers enter the eyeball and distribute to the sphincter pupillae muscle (for pupillary constriction) and to the smooth muscle fibers of the ciliary muscle (for thickening of the lens for near vision)
   b. Fibers from the cells of the oculomotor nucleus also enter the oculomotor nerve (as somatic motor fibers [SE])
      (1) These fibers enter the orbit and innervate the skeletal muscle fibers of the medial rectus muscle (for convergence of the eyeball)

Hearing

1. Receptors
   a. Inner and outer hair cells of the spiral organ located in the cochlear duct of the cochlea
2. Peripheral processes of bipolar cell bodies (dendrites)
   a. Short peripheral processes of the bipolar cells of the spiral ganglion
3. Cell bodies of the first-order neurons
   a. Bipolar cells of the spiral ganglion located in the modiolus of the cochlea
4. Central processes of bipolar cell bodies (axons)
   a. Converge to form the cochlear part of the vestibulocochlear nerve (VIII)
   b. Leave the petrous part of the temporal bone through the internal acoustic meatus
   c. Enter the pons-medulla junction by way of the vestibulocochlear nerve (VIII)
5. First synapse
   a. Dorsal and ventral cochlear nuclei of the lower pons—upper medulla
6. Course of axons of the second-order neurons
   a. Most (but not all) of the fibers cross to the contralateral side of the pons in the trapezoid body (and other parts of the pons)
   b. Enter the *lateral lemniscus*
   c. The lateral lemniscus ascends through the brainstem and ends (mainly) in the inferior colliculus
   d. As the lateral lemniscus is formed and ascends through the brainstem, fibers leave and enter it—going to and coming from the nuclei of the trapezoid body, the superior olivary nucleus, and the nucleus of the lateral lemniscus
   e. In addition to those fibers that cross in the trapezoid body, some fibers cross the midline in between the two nuclei of the lateral lemnisci (in the upper pons), others cross in the commissure of the inferior colliculi, and still others remain uncrossed and ascend in the ipsilateral lateral lemniscus
      (1) Therefore, in some cases these second-order neurons may be third- or fourth-order neurons by the time they reach the inferior colliculus

7. Second synapse
   a. Mainly in the inferior colliculus of the midbrain
   b. As mentioned above, also in the nuclei of the trapezoid body, the superior olivary nucleus, and the nucleus of the lateral lemniscus
8. Course of axons of the third-order neurons
   a. Enter the *brachium of the inferior colliculus*
9. Third synapse
   a. Medial geniculate body of the thalamus
10. Course of axons of the fourth-order neurons
    a. Enter the *geniculocortical fibers* (or *auditory radiations*)
    b. Pass through the sublenticular part of the internal capsule
    c. End in the primary auditory cortex (area 41) and the secondary auditory cortex (area 42) on the transverse temporal gyri of the temporal lobe
    d. Area 22, on the superior temporal gyrus of the temporal lobe, is the *auditory association area* and must be intact if you are to interpret what you hear

Equilibrium

1. Receptors
   a. Hair cells of the crista ampullaris located in the ampulla of each semicircular duct—for dynamic equilibrium (angular acceleration)
   b. Hair cells of the macula utriculi and the macula sacculi located in the utricle and the saccule of the vestibule of the inner ear—for static equilibrium (changes in gravitational forces, linear acceleration, and the position of the head in space)
2. Peripheral processes of bipolar cell bodies (dendrites)
   a. Short peripheral processes of the bipolar cells of the vestibular ganglion
3. Cell bodies of the first-order neurons
   a. Bipolar cells of the vestibular ganglion located in the internal acoustic meatus
4. Central processes of bipolar cell bodies (axons)
   a. Form the vestibular part of the vestibulocochlear nerve (VIII)
   b. Leave the petrous part of the temporal bone through the internal acoustic meatus
   c. Enter the pons-medulla junction by way of the vestibulocochlear nerve (VIII)
   d. *Some* (not most) of the fibers enter the ipsilateral side of the cerebellum and end in the cortex of the uvula, flocculus, and nodulus
5. First synapse
   a. Superior, lateral, medial, and inferior vestibular nuclei of the upper medulla–lower pons

6. Course of axons of the second-order neurons
   a. Fibers from the inferior and medial vestibular nuclei enter the cerebellum and end in the nodulus, flocculus, uvula, and the fastigial nucleus
      (1) The fastigial nuclei and portions of the cortex of the cerebellar vermis send efferent fibers to the lateral vestibular nucleus
   b. Fibers from the lateral vestibular nucleus enter the *vestibulospinal tract,* which distributes throughout the length of the spinal cord ipsilaterally, facilitating reflex activity and muscle tonus
      (1) This tract helps control body movements in response to vestibular stimuli
   c. Fibers from all of the vestibular nuclei enter the *medial longitudinal fasciculus* (MLF). These fibers are both crossed and uncrossed, and many split into ascending and descending branches
      (1) Descending vestibular fibers in the MLF arise from the medial vestibular nucleus (perhaps also the lateral and inferior nuclei)
         (a) They descend through the medulla and enter the anterior funiculus of the spinal cord
         (b) They distribute only to the cervical spinal cord
         (c) This tract helps control head and arm movements in response to vestibular stimuli
      (2) Ascending vestibular fibers in the MLF arise from all the vestibular nuclei. They mainly project to the nuclei of the extraocular muscles (i.e., the oculomotor, trochlear, and abducent nuclei). Thus, the main function of these fibers is to provide vestibular, and probably cerebellar, input into the functioning of the extraocular muscles
         (a) There are pathways controlling the horizontal movement of the eyes subsequent to turning the head horizontally, and the vertical movement of the eyes subsequent to turning the head vertically (the nonoptic reflex eye movement system)
         (b) Both of these pathways enable you to focus on a point as you turn your head

Motor Pathways

SOMATIC EFFERENTS AND SPECIAL VISCERAL EFFERENTS TO THE HEAD AND NECK (CORTICONUCLEAR [CORTICOBULBAR] FIBERS OF THE PYRAMIDAL TRACT)

Eye Movements (SE)

The pathways that control eye movements are varied and complex. Gay and his colleagues described five different eye movement systems: the saccadic system (for rapid, voluntary eye movements), the smooth pursuit system (for following or tracking eye movements), the vergence system (for convergence or divergence), the nonoptic reflex system (for reflex eye movements in response to vestibular or neck receptor stimuli), and the position maintenance system (for maintaining gaze fixation on a target). The pathways mediating these various types of eye movement are known to variable degrees. Those pathways controlling conjugate eye movements (saccades, pursuit, and nonoptic reflexes) are known in greater detail than those governing the vergence system and the position maintenance system. I will describe only the saccadic system and the smooth pursuit system here, since these are the systems most commonly tested clinically and the systems about which we know the most. The nonoptic reflex system was alluded to previously (although not fully described) in the section on equilibrium.

The Saccadic System (Rapid Eye Movements, Voluntary Eye Movements)

There are two pathways that govern voluntary, or rapid, eye movements (saccades), one for horizontal eye movements and one for vertical eye movements. These are outlined separately below.
A. Pathway for voluntary horizontal conjugate eye movements
  1. Location of upper motor neuron cell bodies
    a. Motor cortex for voluntary eye movements (frontal eye field, area 8) located mainly on the middle frontal gyrus of the frontal lobe
    b. Horizontal eye movements are mediated by the contralateral frontal eye field (i.e., horizontal conjugate eye movements to the right are controlled by the left frontal lobe, and vice versa)

  2. Course of axons of the upper motor neurons
    a. Fibers pass through the corona radiata
    b. Pass through the anterior limb of the internal capsule
    c. Pass into the reticular formation of the midbrain
    d. Between the oculomotor and trochlear nuclei of the midbrain, the fibers cross the midline and continue to descend through the reticular formation of the midbrain and the pons
    e. In the lower third of the pons, the fibers pass into the *pontine center for horizontal conjugate gaze,* which is located in the paramedian pontine reticular formation near the abducent nucleus
      (1) The neurons of the pontine horizontal gaze center send their axons into the ipsilateral abducent nucleus and into the contralateral medial longitudinal fasciculus (MLF)
      (2) The axons that enter the contralateral MLF ascend to the part of the oculomotor nucleus that controls the medial rectus muscle
  3. Location of lower motor neuron cell bodies
    a. Abducent nucleus
    b. The part of the oculomotor nucleus (contralateral to the abducent nucleus) that controls the medial rectus muscle
  4. Course of axons of the lower motor neurons
    a. Enter the abducent nerve (VI) and travel with it into the orbit
    b. Enter the contralateral oculomotor nerve (III) and travel with it into the orbit
  5. Structures innervated
    a. Lateral rectus muscle via the abducent nerve
    b. Contralateral medial rectus muscle via the oculomotor nerve

B. Pathway for voluntary vertical conjugate eye movements
  1. Location of upper motor neuron cell bodies
    a. Motor cortex for voluntary eye movements (frontal eye field, area 8) located mainly on the middle frontal gyrus of the frontal lobe
    b. Vertical eye movements are mediated by simultaneous activity of both frontal eye fields; therefore, unilateral supranuclear (upper motor neuron) lesions will not affect vertical eye movements
  2. Course of axons of the upper motor neurons
    a. Fibers pass through the corona radiata (bilaterally)
    b. Pass through the anterior limb of the internal capsule
    c. Crossed and uncrossed fibers pass into the *pretectal center for vertical conjugate gaze* near the cerebral aqueduct in the pretectal region of the midbrain
      (1) The neurons of the pretectal vertical gaze center project their axons diffusely and bilaterally into the oculomotor and trochlear nuclei of the midbrain
  3. Location of lower motor neuron cell bodies
    a. All parts of the oculomotor nuclei except those that innervate the medial rectus muscles
    b. Trochlear nuclei
  4. Course of axons of the lower motor neurons
    a. Enter the oculomotor nerves (III) and travel with them into the orbits
    b. Cross the midline in the tectum of the midbrain, enter the trochlear nerves (IV), and travel with them into the orbits
  5. Structures innervated
    a. Superior and inferior rectus muscles and the inferior oblique muscles via the oculomotor nerves
    b. Superior oblique muscles via the trochlear nerves

The Smooth Pursuit System (Following, or Tracking, Eye Movements)

There are also two pathways that control following, or pursuit, eye movements; again, one for horizontal eye movements and one for vertical eye movements.
A. Pathway for horizontal pursuit eye movements
  1. Location of upper motor neuron cell bodies
    a. Anterior occipital lobe (areas 18 and 19)
    b. Horizontal pursuit movements are mediated by the contralateral occipital lobe (i.e., horizontal pursuit movements to the right are controlled by the left occipital lobe, and vice versa)
  2. Course of axons of the upper motor neurons
    a. Fibers pass through the retrolenticular part of the posterior limb of the internal capsule and perhaps also through the pulvinar of the thalamus
    b. Pass into the reticular formation of the midbrain
    c. Between the oculomotor and trochlear nuclei of the midbrain, the fibers cross the midline and continue to descend through the reticular formation of the midbrain and the pons
    d. In the lower third of the pons, the fibers pass into the *pontine center for horizontal conjugate gaze,* which is located in the paramedian pontine reticular formation near the abducent nucleus
      (1) The neurons of the pontine horizontal gaze center send their axons into the ipsilateral abducent nucleus and into the contralateral medial longitudinal fasciculus (MLF)
      (2) The axons that enter the contralateral MLF ascend to the part of the oculomotor nucleus that controls the medial rectus muscle
  3. Location of lower motor neuron cell bodies
    a. Abducent nucleus
    b. The part of the oculomotor nucleus (contralateral to the abducent nucleus) that controls the medial rectus muscle
  4. Course of axons of the lower motor neurons
    a. Enter the abducent nerve (VI) and travel with it into the orbit
    b. Enter the contralateral oculomotor nerve (III) and travel with it into the orbit
  5. Structures innervated
    a. Lateral rectus muscle via the abducent nerve
    b. Contralateral medial rectus muscle via the oculomotor nerve

B. Pathway for vertical pursuit eye movements
   1. Location of upper motor neuron cell bodies
      a. Anterior occipital lobe (areas 18 and 19)
      b. Vertical pursuit movements are mediated by simultaneous activity of both occipital lobes
   2. Course of axons of the upper motor neurons
      a. Fibers pass through the retrolenticular part of the posterior limb of the internal capsule and perhaps also through the pulvinar of the thalamus (bilaterally)
      b. Crossed and uncrossed fibers pass into the *pretectal center for vertical conjugate gaze* near the cerebral aqueduct in the pretectal region of the midbrain
         (1) The neurons of the pretectal vertical gaze center project their axons diffusely and bilaterally into the oculomotor and trochlear nuclei of the midbrain
   3. Location of lower motor neuron cell bodies
      a. All parts of the oculomotor nuclei except those that innervate the medial rectus muscles
      b. Trochlear nuclei
   4. Course of axons of the lower motor neurons
      a. Enter the oculomotor nerves (III) and travel with them into the orbits
      b. Cross the midline in the tectum of the midbrain, enter the trochlear nerves (IV), and travel with them into the orbits
   5. Structures innervated
      a. Superior and inferior rectus muscles and the inferior oblique muscles via the oculomotor nerves
      b. Superior oblique muscles via the trochlear nerves

Head and Neck Movements Controlled by Special Visceral Efferent Neurons

   1. Location of upper motor neuron cell bodies
      a. Face region of the motor cortex (area 4) located on the precentral gyrus of the frontal lobe
      b. Also areas 6, 3, 1, and 2
   2. Course of axons of the upper motor neurons
      a. Pass through the corona radiata
      b. Pass through the third quarter of the posterior limb of the internal capsule
      c. Pass through the medial side of the middle three-fifths of the crus cerebri of the midbrain
      d. Pass through the dispersed pyramidal tract bundles of the pons
      e. In the middle third of the pons, *mainly* crossed (but also some uncrossed) fibers pass into the motor nucleus of the trigeminal nerve (V)
      f. In the lower third of the pons, crossed fibers pass into the anterior part of the facial nucleus (which innervates the lower facial muscles), and crossed and uncrossed fibers pass into the posterior part of the facial nucleus (which innervates the upper facial muscles)
      g. In the medulla, the *pyramidal tract* reunites and forms the pyramids of the medulla
      h. In the medulla, crossed and uncrossed fibers pass into the nucleus ambiguus
   3. Location of lower motor neuron cell bodies
      a. Motor nucleus of V
      b. Facial nucleus—anterior and posterior parts
      c. Nucleus ambiguus
      d. Accessory nucleus—This is the nucleus of the spinal part of the accessory nerve (XI), which is located in the first 5 segments of the cervical spinal cord. These cell bodies synapse with mainly uncrossed upper motor neurons
   4. Course of axons of the lower motor neurons
      a. Fibers distribute with the mandibular division of the trigeminal nerve (V)
      b. Fibers distribute with the facial nerve (VII)
      c. Fibers distribute with the glossopharyngeal nerve (IX), the vagus nerve (X), and the cranial part of the accessory nerve (XI)
      d. Fibers distribute with the spinal part of the accessory nerve (XI)
   5. Structures innervated
      a. Muscles of mastication; tensor veli palatini, tensor tympani, mylohyoid, and anterior digastric muscles via the trigeminal nerve (mandibular division)
      b. Lower facial muscles (supplied by fibers arising in the anterior part of the facial nucleus), upper facial muscles (from the posterior part of the facial nucleus), stapedius, stylohyoid, and posterior digastric muscles via the facial nerve

c. Stylopharyngeus via the glossopharyngeal nerve; muscles of the soft palate, pharynx, esophagus, and larynx via the vagus nerve (the cranial part of the accessory nerve may also supply the muscles of the larynx and the pharynx)
d. Sternocleidomastoid and trapezius muscles via the spinal part of the accessory nerve

Tongue Movements (SE)

1. Location of upper motor neuron cell bodies
   a. Tongue region of the motor cortex (area 4) located on the precentral gyrus of the frontal lobe
   b. Also areas 6, 3, 1, and 2
2. Course of axons of the upper motor neurons
   a. Pass through the corona radiata
   b. Pass through the third quarter of the posterior limb of the internal capsule
   c. Pass through the medial side of the middle three-fifths of the crus cerebri of the midbrain
   d. Pass through the dispersed pyramidal tract bundles of the pons
   e. In the medulla, the *pyramidal tract* reunites and forms the pyramids of the medulla
   f. In the lower medulla, *mainly* crossed fibers pass into the hypoglossal nucleus
3. Location of lower motor neuron cell bodies
   a. Hypoglossal nucleus
4. Course of axons of the lower motor neurons
   a. Fibers distribute with the hypoglossal nerve (XII)
5. Structures innervated
   a. Intrinsic and extrinsic muscles of the tongue via the hypoglossal nerve

SOMATIC EFFERENTS TO THE BODY

Pyramidal System (Corticospinal Fibers of the Pyramidal Tract)

1. Location of upper motor neuron cell bodies
   a. Upper limb, trunk, and lower limb regions of the motor cortex (area 4) located on the precentral gyrus of the frontal lobe
   b. Also areas 6, 3, 1, and 2
2. Course of axons of the upper motor neurons
   a. Enter the *corticospinal part of the pyramidal tract* (the other part of the pyramidal tract being the *corticonuclear* [or *corticobulbar*] *fibers,* outlined on the preceding pages)
   b. Pass through the corona radiata
   c. Pass through the third quarter of the posterior limb of the internal capsule
   d. Pass through the middle and lateral side of the middle three-fifths of the crus cerebri of the midbrain
   e. Pass through the dispersed pyramidal tract bundles of the pons
   f. In the medulla, the *pyramidal tract* reunites and forms the pyramids of the medulla
   g. In the low medulla, the fibers to the upper limb (first) and the lower limb (lower in the medulla) cross to the contralateral side of the body in the pyramidal decussation and form the *lateral corticospinal* (or *pyramidal*) *tract* of the spinal cord
      (1) 75% to 90% of the corticospinal fibers cross in the pyramidal decussation
      (2) Many of the fibers to the trunk muscles remain uncrossed and form the *anterior corticospinal* (or *pyramidal*) *tract* of the spinal cord
   h. The two corticospinal tracts then descend in the lateral and anterior funiculi of the spinal cord to the level of their synapses
   i. In the cervical cord, upper limb fibers leave the lateral corticospinal tract and pass into the gray matter of the spinal cord
   j. In the thoracic cord mainly, but also in the cervical and lumbar cords, the trunk fibers leave the anterior corticospinal tract, cross to the contralateral side of the cord in the white commissure, and pass into the gray matter of the spinal cord
   k. In the lumbar and sacral regions of the cord, lower limb fibers leave the lateral corticospinal tract and pass into the gray matter of the cord
   l. Some upper motor neurons synapse directly with the alpha motor neurons of the anterior horn of the spinal cord. Others, however (as in the brainstem), synapse with internuncial neurons, which in turn synapse with the alpha motor neurons of the anterior horn

3. Location of lower motor neuron cell bodies
   a. Alpha motor neurons located in the nuclei of the medial (for trunk muscles) and lateral (for upper and lower limb muscles) divisions of the anterior horn of the spinal cord
4. Course of axons of the lower motor neurons
   a. Leave the spinal cord through the ventral roots
   b. Pass into the spinal nerves
   c. Pass into the dorsal rami (only fibers to trunk muscles) and the ventral rami (upper limb, lower limb, and trunk fibers) of the spinal nerves
   d. Distribute with all of the muscular branches of the dorsal and ventral rami of the spinal nerves
5. Structures innervated
   a. Skeletal muscles of the upper and lower limbs and the trunk

Extrapyramidal System

The extrapyramidal motor system is the name given to the somatic efferent system, which consists of pathways other than those of the pyramidal tract. Functionally, it is concerned with the grosser, more automatic, voluntary movements (as well as postural adjustments); as opposed to the fine, isolated, versatile movements controlled by the pyramidal system. The extrapyramidal system is intimately related to the basal ganglia and, secondarily, to certain brainstem nuclei (e.g., the subthalamic nucleus, the substantia nigra, the red nucleus, and the brainstem reticular formation). To simplify matters, I will begin the description of the extrapyramidal system with the basal ganglia. However, you should keep in mind that the basal ganglia receive afferent fibers from the cerebral cortex (corticostriate fibers), from the centromedian nucleus of the thalamus (thalamostriate fibers), and from the substantia nigra (nigrostriate fibers). These afferent fibers, along with their afferents, are part of the elaborate feedback mechanism that is continually controlling this system.

1. Afferent input into the basal ganglia
   a. Most input comes into the caudate nucleus and the putamen, and most output is via the globus pallidus
   b. Corticostriate fibers
      (1) Essentially the entire cerebral cortex sends fibers into the caudate nucleus and the putamen
   c. Thalamostriate fibers
   d. Nigrostriate fibers
   e. Short internuncial neurons project from the caudate nucleus and the putamen to the globus pallidus, where they synapse with the "upper motor neurons"
2. Location of primary upper motor neuron cell bodies
   a. Cerebral cortex
   b. Globus pallidus

3. Course of axons of the primary upper motor neurons
   a. Fibers descend to the superior collicular level of the midbrain and pass into the red nucleus
   b. Fibers from the globus pallidus enter the *ansa lenticularis* and the *lenticular fasciculus,* which may send a small number of fibers into the midbrain (tegmentum, red nucleus?)
   c. Most of the fibers of the ansa lenticularis and the lenticular fasciculus pass medially and then curve upward and backward to enter the *thalamic fasciculus*
      (1) The thalamic fasciculus projects to the ventral anterior and ventral lateral nuclei of the thalamus
      (2) These two thalamic nuclei, in turn, project to the motor and premotor cortices (areas 4 and 6); thereby completing an important feedback loop for the control of motor activity
4. Location of secondary upper motor neuron cell bodies
   a. Red nucleus of the midbrain
   b. Reticular formation of the midbrain (probably other regions of the brainstem as well)
   c. Other areas of the brainstem (e.g., superior colliculus, vestibular nuclei)
5. Course of axons of the secondary upper motor neurons
   a. Fibers from the red nucleus cross the midline and enter the *rubrospinal tract*
   b. The tract descends through the brainstem and enters the lateral funiculus of the spinal cord
   c. The tract descends through the spinal cord located just anterior to the lateral corticospinal tract
   d. Fibers pass out of the tract and into the gray matter of the cord, where they synapse with internuncial neurons
      (1) The internuncial neurons synapse either with alpha motor neurons (inhibitory) or with gamma motor neurons in the anterior horn of the spinal cord
   e. There are other descending extrapyramidal tracts (e.g., reticulospinal, vestibulospinal, tectospinal) which will not be considered here
6. Location of lower motor neuron cell bodies
   a. Alpha and gamma motor neurons located in the anterior horn of the spinal cord
7. Course of axons of the lower motor neurons
   a. Enter the ventral roots, the spinal nerves, and the muscular branches of the dorsal and ventral rami of the spinal nerves
8. Structures innervated
   a. Skeletal muscles of the body for gross, automatic, and postural movements

CEREBELLAR CONNECTIONS

Although the cerebellum functions at an unconscious, involuntary level, it is an extremely important part of the brain with respect to motor functioning. It receives sensory input from all of the general and special senses and has efferent connections (direct or indirect) with most parts of the central nervous system. The cerebellum receives most of its afferent fibers through the inferior and middle cerebellar peduncles, whereas most of its efferent fibers leave by way of the superior and inferior cerebellar peduncles. The cerebellum is primarily concerned with three types of functional mechanisms: those that influence and maintain equilibrium, those that regulate muscle tone, and those that regulate the timing and precision (i.e., coordination) of somatic motor activity. Therefore, although there are several pathways and patterns of cerebellar connections, I will describe only the three main groups of connections by which the cerebellum exerts its influence.

Vestibular (Archicerebellar) Connections

1. Input
   a. Primary (directly from the vestibulocochlear nerve) and secondary (from the vestibular nuclei) vestibular fibers enter the cerebellum through the *inferior cerebellar peduncle* and end as the mossy fibers of the archicerebellum (or *flocculonodular lobe)*
   b. The mossy fibers synapse with granule cells, which in turn synapse with Purkinje cells in the cerebellar cortex
2. Output
   a. The Purkinje cells of the archicerebellum project to the fastigial nucleus of the cerebellum
   b. The cells of the fastigial nucleus send their axons out of the cerebellum mainly through the *inferior cerebellar peduncle*
   c. These fibers end in the vestibular nuclei (and the brainstem reticular formation)
3. Function
   a. Maintenance of equilibrium
   b. Maintenance of posture and balance of the trunk

Spinal (Paleocerebellar) Connections

1. Input
   a. Sensory information (particularly unconscious proprioception from muscle spindles and neurotendinous organs) carried in the *anterior* and *posterior spinocerebellar tracts* and the *external arcuate fibers* (also the spinoolivary to olivocerebellar tracts and the spinoreticular to reticulocerebellar tracts) enters the cerebellum through the *inferior cerebellar peduncle*
   b. Within the cerebellum, these fibers end as the mossy fibers of the *paleocerebellum* (or *anterior lobe)*
   c. The mossy fibers synapse with granule cells, which in turn synapse with Purkinje cells
2. Output
   a. The Purkinje cells of the paleocerebellum project to the fastigial nucleus
   b. The cells of the fastigial nucleus send their axons out of the cerebellum mainly through the *inferior cerebellar peduncle*
   c. These fibers end in the brainstem reticular formation (and the vestibular nuclei) and thereby influence descending tracts of the extrapyramidal system
3. Function
   a. Regulation of muscle tone by facilitating spinal reflexes via the gamma efferent system
   b. Maintenance of posture and balance of the limbs

Cortical (Neocerebellar) Connections

1. Input
   a. Information from the cerebral cortex (especially concerning somatic motor functioning) descends through the midbrain in the *pyramidal tract,* the *frontopontine tract,* and the *temporoparietooccipitopontine tract*
   b. In the pons, these tracts synapse with pontine nuclei in the ipsilateral side of the ventral part (or basis) of the pons
   c. The axons of these cells form the pontocerebellar fibers, which cross to the contralateral side of the pons and enter the *middle cerebellar peduncle*
   d. These fibers enter the cerebellum through the middle cerebellar peduncle and end as the mossy fibers of the *neocerebellum* (or *posterior lobe*)
   e. The mossy fibers synapse with granule cells, which in turn synapse with Purkinje cells
2. Output
   a. The Purkinje cells of the neocerebellum project to the dentate nucleus of the cerebellum
   b. The cells of the dentate nucleus send their axons into the *dentatorubrothalamic tract,* which passes out of the cerebellum through the *superior cerebellar peduncle*
   c. The dentatorubrothalamic tract crosses to the contralateral side of the brainstem in the decussation of the superior cerebellar peduncle at the inferior collicular level of the midbrain
   d. Some of the fibers of the tract synapse with cells in the red nucleus, while others pass around the red nucleus without synapsing
   e. The tract, including fibers from the red nucleus, continues to ascend and ends in the ventral lateral nucleus of the thalamus
   f. Fibers from the ventral lateral nucleus of the thalamus project to the (original ipsilateral) motor cortex (area 4 and maybe area 6); thereby completing another important feedback loop for the control of motor activity
3. Function
   a. Regulation of the timing and precision (i.e., coordination) of discrete limb movements (or somatic motor activity)

III
ATLAS OF THE BRAIN
AND SPINAL CORD

SURFACE VIEWS OF THE BRAIN

Figure 2. Lateral View of Brain, Arachnoid and Pia Mater Intact (×1)

A. Frontal pole of cerebral hemisphere
B. Frontal lobe
C. Parietal lobe
D. Occipital lobe
E. Occipital pole
F. Temporal pole
G. Temporal lobe
H. Small piece of dura mater
 I. Superficial cerebral veins emptying into the superior sagittal sinus
J. Cerebellum
K. Pons
L. Medulla

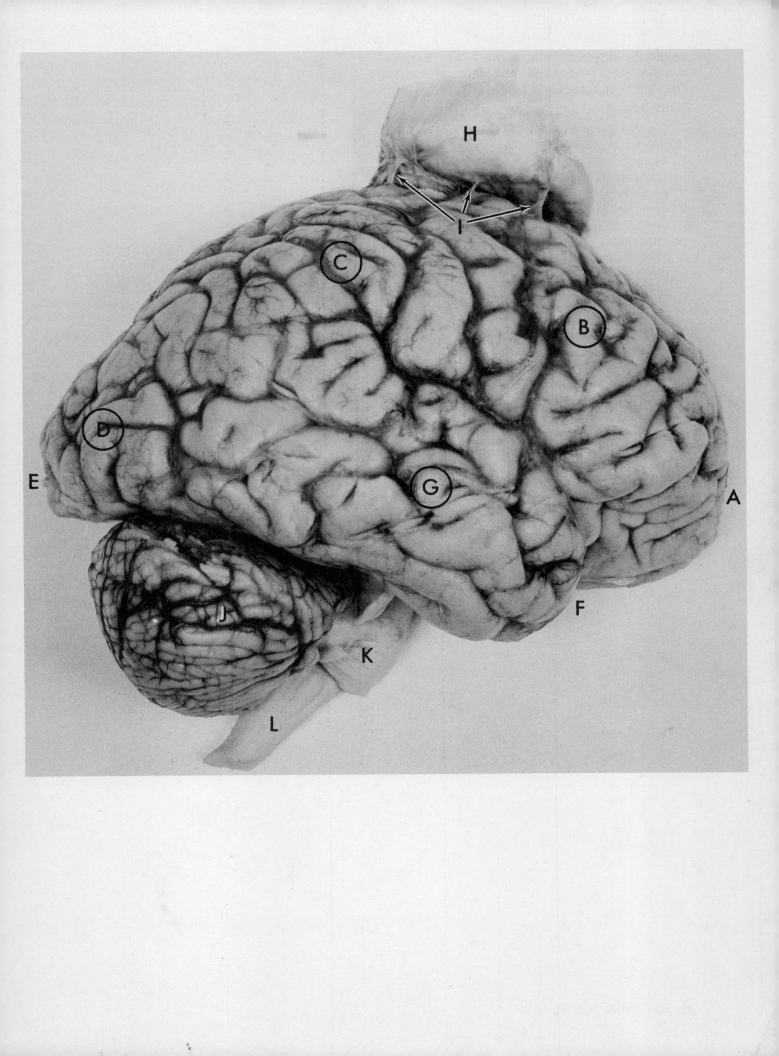

Figure 3. Superior View of the Brain, Arachnoid and Pia Mater Intact on Right Cerebral Hemisphere and Removed from Left (×1)

A. Small piece of dura mater
B. Arachnoid granulations
C. Longitudinal cerebral fissure
D. Superior frontal gyrus
E. Superior frontal sulcus
F. Precentral sulcus
G. Precentral gyrus
H. Central sulcus
I. Postcentral gyrus
J. Postcentral sulcus
K. Marginal ramus of cingulate sulcus
L. Occipital lobe

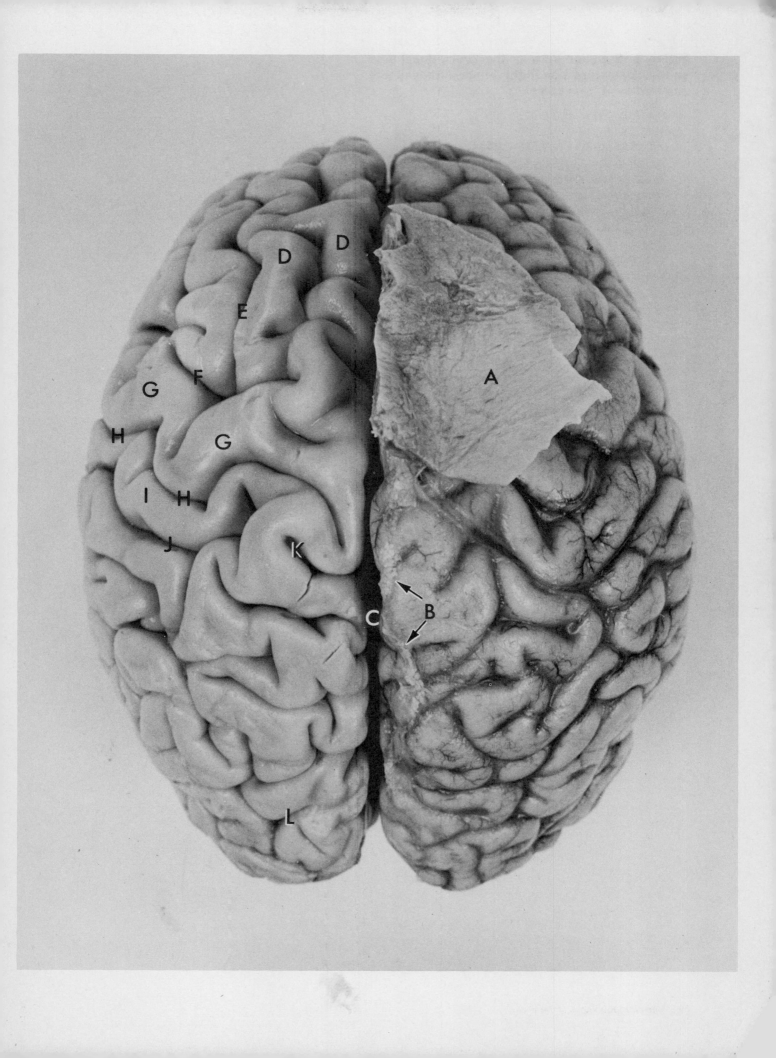

Figure 4. Base of the Brain Showing Arterial Supply and Cranial Nerves. Anteroinferior View (×1.5)

A. Olfactory sulcus
B. Olfactory bulb
C. Olfactory tract
D. Anterior cerebral artery (notice difference in size between right and left)
E. Anterior communicating artery
F. Posterior cerebral artery
G. Oculomotor nerve (III)
H. Superior cerebellar artery (double on the right)
I. Basilar artery
J. Trigeminal nerve (V)
K. Facial nerve (VII)
L. Vestibulocochlear nerve (VIII)
M. Glossopharyngeal (IX), vagus (X), and cranial part of accessory (XI) nerves
N. Vertebral artery
O. Posterior inferior cerebellar artery

Can you locate:

Internal carotid artery
Middle cerebral artery
Posterior communicating artery
Anterior inferior cerebellar artery
Inferior horn of lateral ventricle

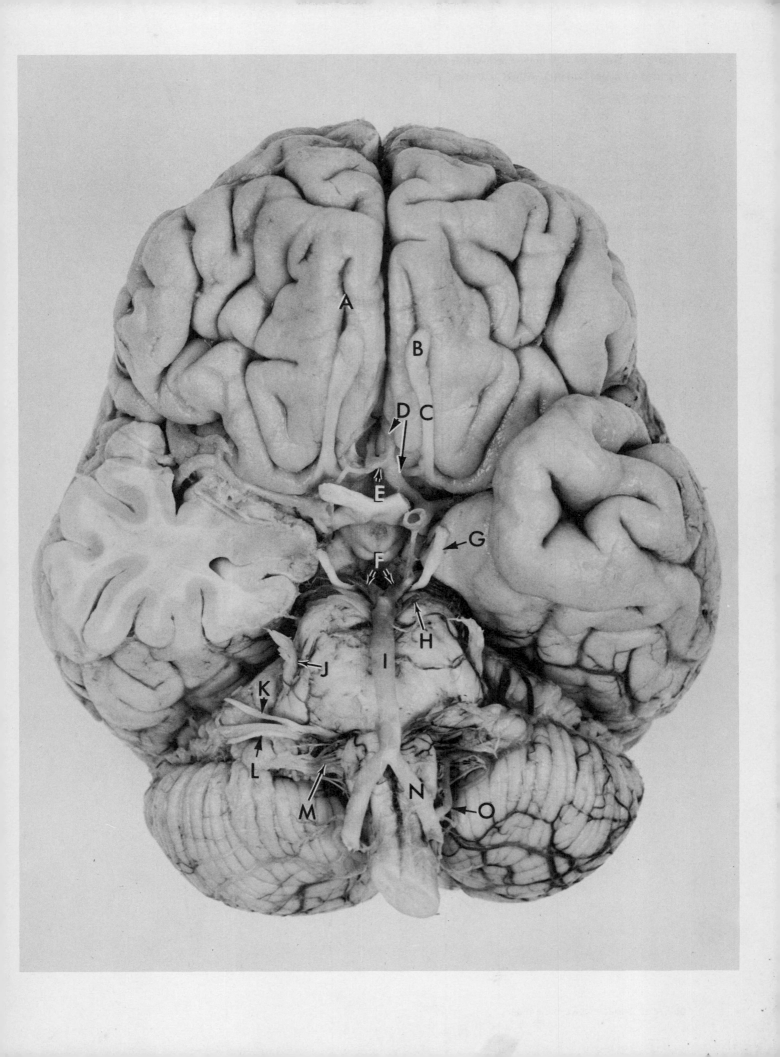

Figure 5. Base of the Brain Showing Arterial Supply and Cranial Nerves. Inferior View (×1.5)

A. Longitudinal cerebral fissure
B. Optic nerve (II)
C. Optic chiasma
D. Optic tract
E. Internal carotid artery
F. Middle cerebral artery (in lateral sulcus)
G. Posterior communicating artery
H. Cut surface of temporal lobe
I. Inferior horn of lateral ventricle

Can you locate:

Anterior cerebral arteries
Anterior communicating artery
Posterior cerebral artery
Oculomotor nerve
Superior cerebellar artery
Basilar artery
Vertebral artery
Posterior inferior cerebellar artery
Facial nerve
Vestibulocochlear nerve

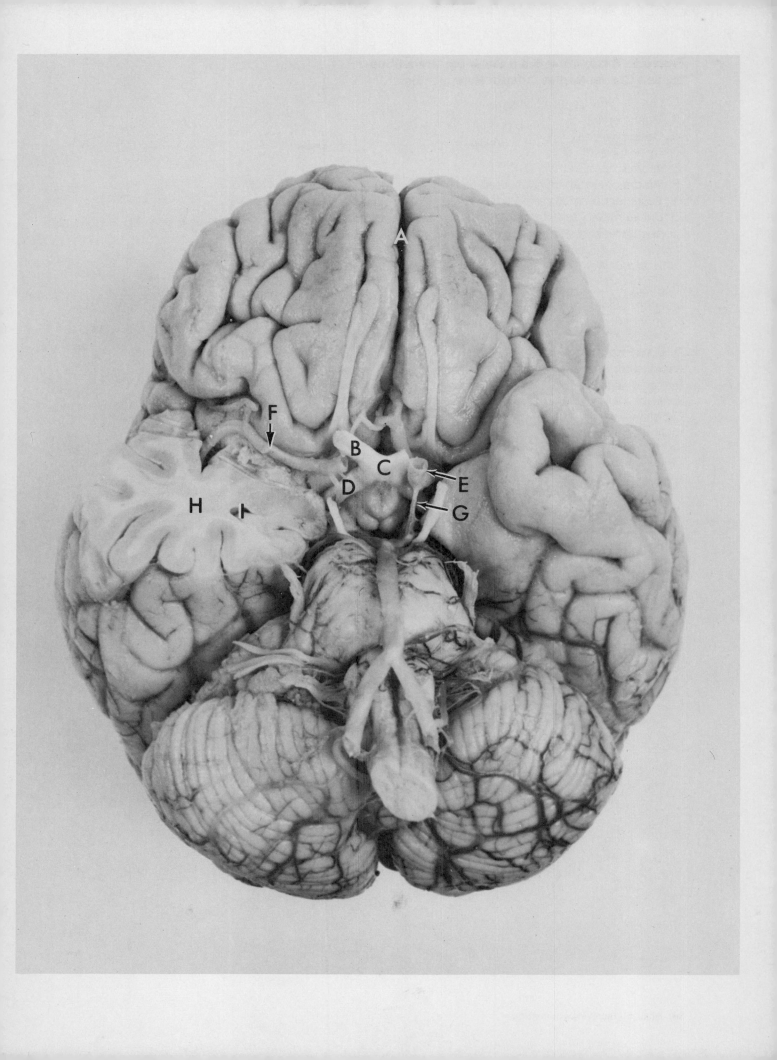

Figure 6. Close-Up of the Base of the Brain Showing the Origin of the Cranial Nerves. Posteroinferior View (×2)

A. Olfactory sulcus
B. Optic nerve (II)
C. Optic chiasma
D. Infundibulum
E. Arachnoid (spanning a sulcus)
F. Oculomotor nerve (III)
G. Facial nerve (VII)
H. Vestibulocochlear nerve (VIII)
I. Stub of abducent nerve (VI)
J. Rootlets of hypoglossal nerve (XII) (emerging from the *anterolateral sulcus* between the *pyramid* ventrally and the *olive* dorsally)

Can you locate:

Olfactory bulb and tract
Gyrus rectus
Mammillary bodies
Basilar artery
Trigeminal nerve
Middle cerebellar peduncle

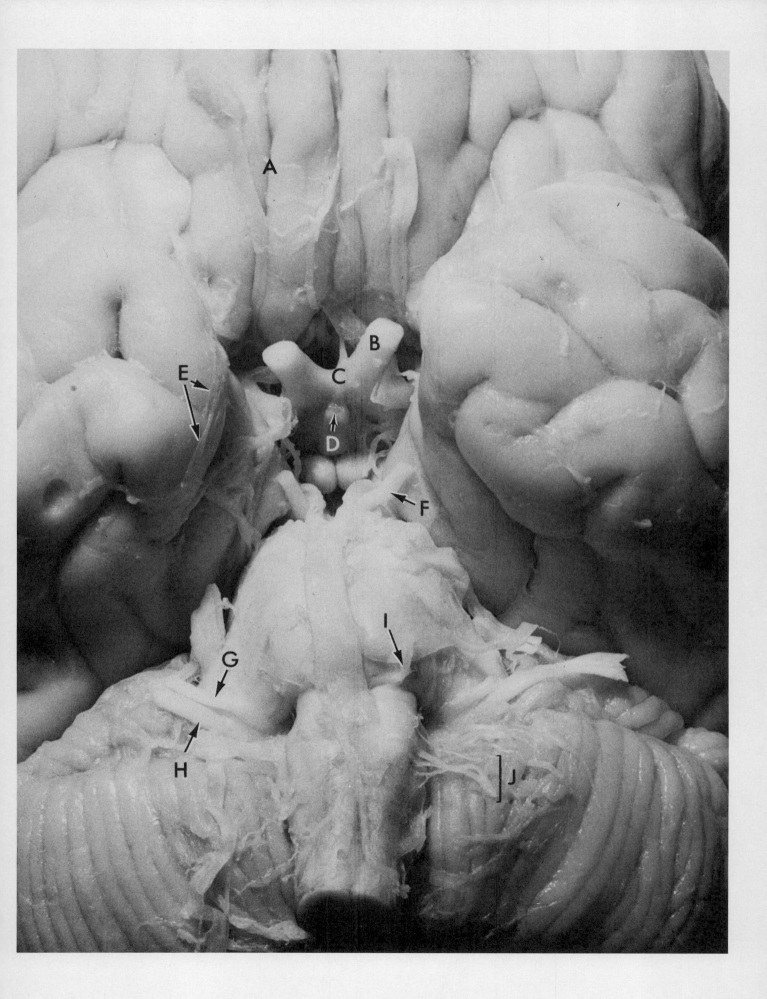

Figure 7. Base of the Brain Showing Cranial Nerves. Arachnoid and Pia Mater Intact on Right Cerebral and Cerebellar Hemispheres and Removed from the Left. Inferior View (×1.5)

A. Straight gyrus (gyrus rectus)
B. Orbital gyri and sulci
C. Olfactory bulb
D. Olfactory tract
E. Oculomotor nerve (III) (emerging from *interpeduncular fossa*)
F. Trochlear nerve (IV) (winding around left *cerebral peduncle*)
G. Pons
H. Trigeminal nerve (V)
 I. Middle cerebellar peduncle
J. Facial nerve (VII)
K. Vestibulocochlear nerve (VIII)
L. Hypoglossal nerve (XII)
M. Flocculus of cerebellum
N. Cerebellar hemisphere

Can you locate:

Longitudinal cerebral fissure
Mammillary bodies
Posterior perforated substance
Pyramid and olive of medulla

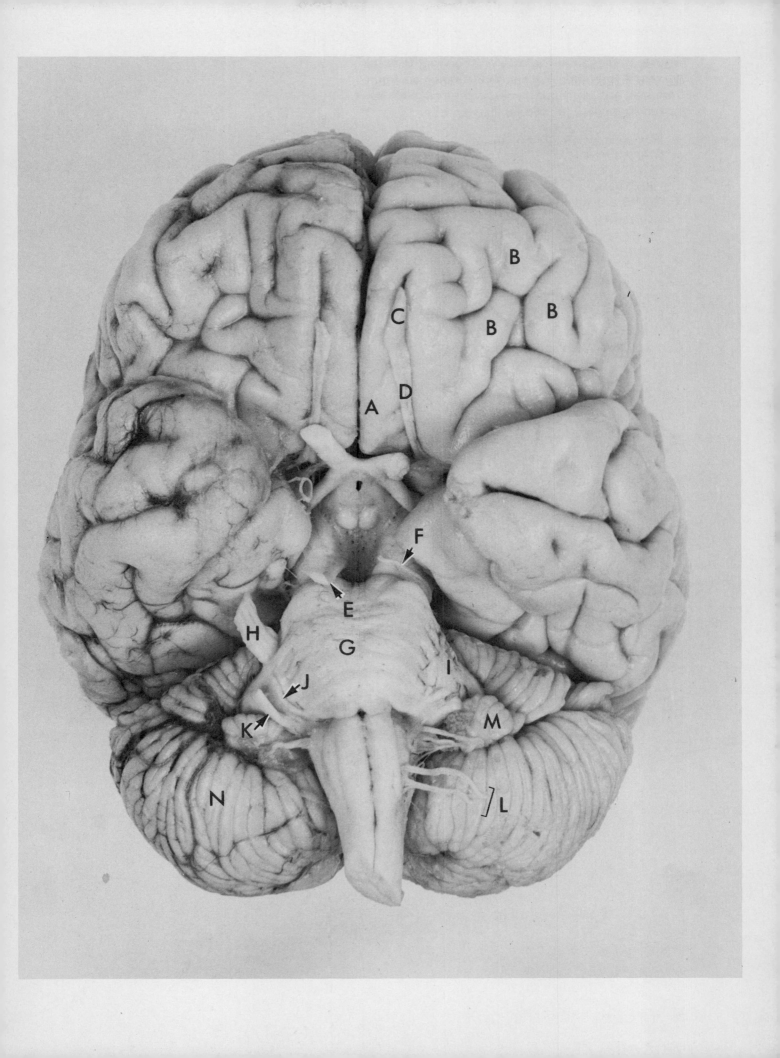

Figure 8. Base of the Brain Showing Cranial Nerves. Arachnoid and Pia Mater Intact on Right Cerebral and Cerebellar Hemispheres and Removed from the Left. Posteroinferior View (×1.5)

A. Longitudinal cerebral fissure
B. Olfactory bulb
C. Olfactory tract
D. Optic nerve (II)
E. Optic chiasma (the hole directly behind the chiasma is in the infundibulum)
F. Optic tract
G. Tuber cinereum
H. Mammillary body
I. Pons
J. Pyramid
K. Olive
L. Collateral sulcus
M. Parahippocampal gyrus
N. Uncus

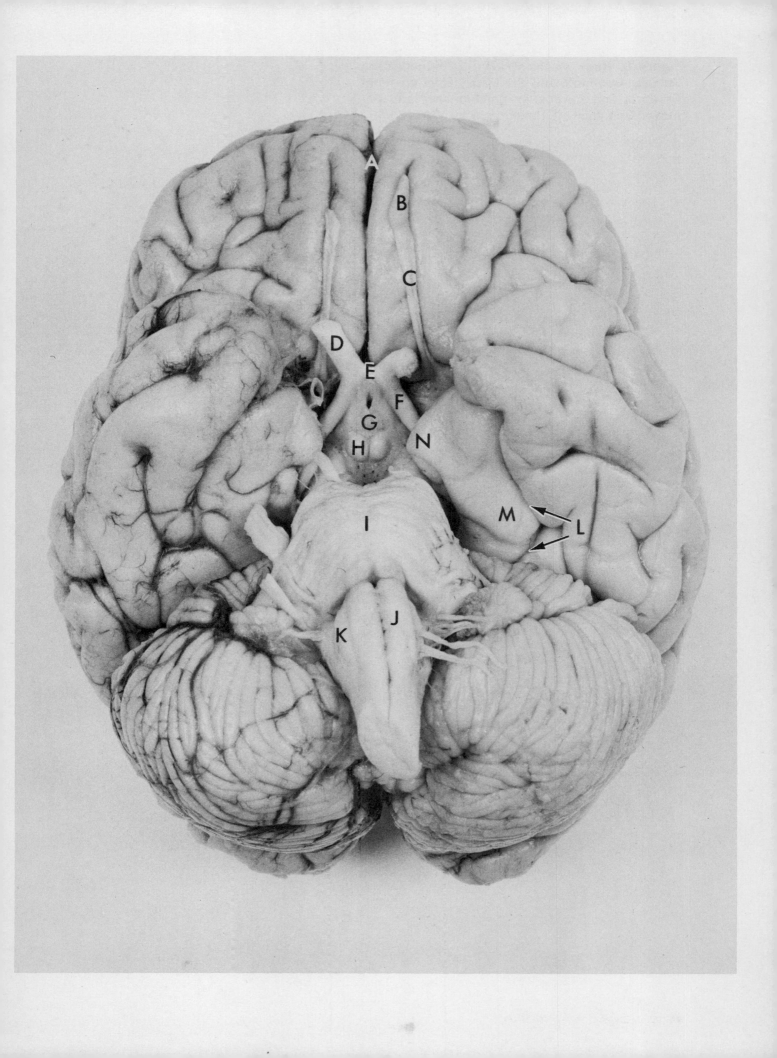

Figure 9. Inferior Surface of the Cerebrum, Brainstem Removed. Posteroinferior View (×1.5)

A. Longitudinal cerebral fissure
B. Optic nerve (II)
C. Infundibulum
D. Midbrain (cut surface)
E. Cerebral aqueduct
F. Inferior colliculus
G. Splenium of corpus callosum
H. Isthmus of cingulate gyrus
I. Calcarine sulcus
J. Lingual gyrus
K. Parahippocampal gyrus
L. Uncus
M. Collateral sulcus
N. Occipitotemporal gyrus
O. Inferior temporal sulcus
P. Inferior temporal gyrus

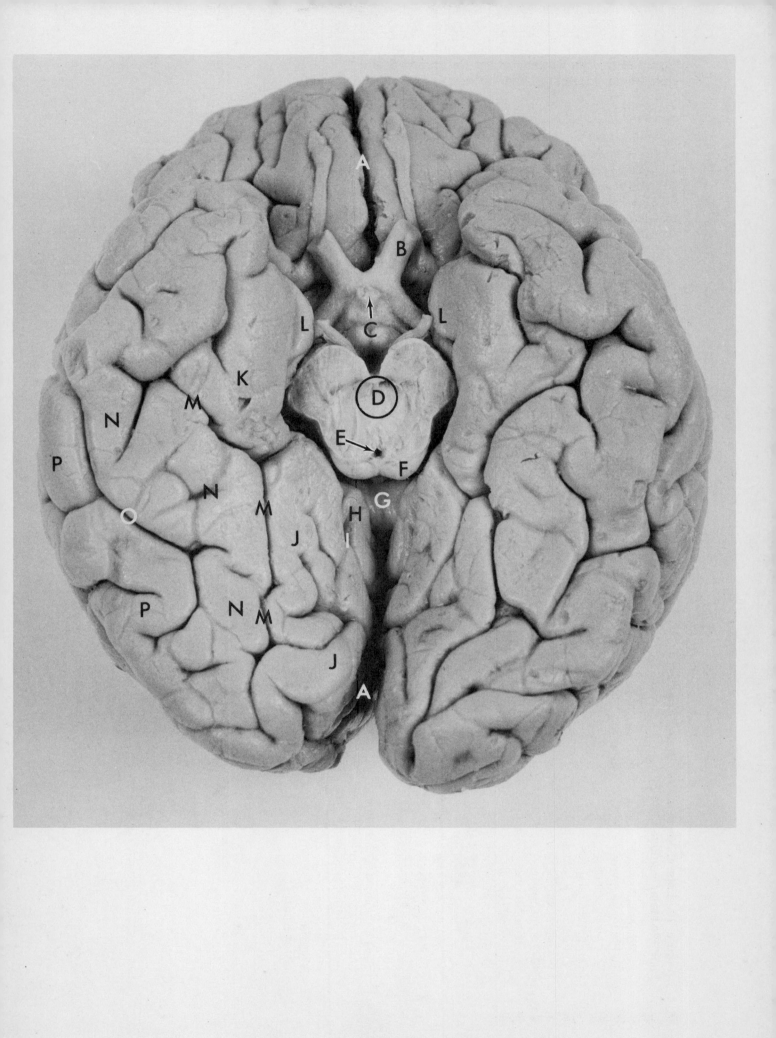

Figure 10. Lateral View of the Brain, Arachnoid and Pia Mater Removed (×1.5)

A. Precentral sulcus
B. Precentral gyrus
C. Central sulcus
D. Postcentral gyrus
E. Postcentral sulcus
F. Supramarginal gyrus
G. Angular gyrus
H. Occipital lobe
I. Lateral sulcus
J. Superior temporal gyrus
K. Superior temporal sulcus
L. Middle temporal gyrus
M. Middle temporal sulcus
N. Inferior temporal gyrus

Can you locate:

Superior, middle, and inferior frontal gyri
Superior and inferior frontal sulci
Frontal, occipital, and temporal poles
Pons
Medulla
Cerebellum

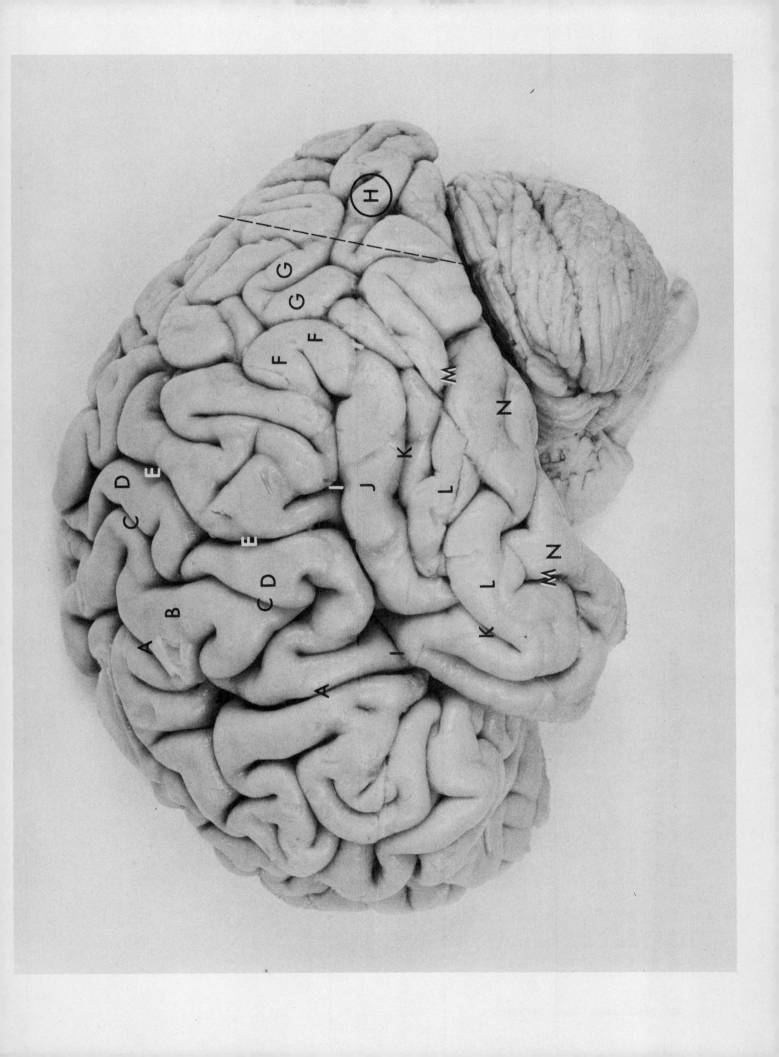

Figure 11. Superolateral View of the Brain, Arach-noid and Pia Mater Removed (×1.5)

A. Superior frontal gyrus
B. Superior frontal sulcus
C. Middle frontal gyrus
D. Inferior frontal sulcus
E. Inferior frontal gyrus
F. Precentral sulcus
G. Precentral gyrus
H. Central sulcus
I. Postcentral gyrus
J. Postcentral sulcus
K. Superior parietal lobule
L. Intraparietal sulcus
M. Inferior parietal lobule
N. Cerebellum

Can you locate:

Marginal ramus of cingulate sulcus
Supramarginal and angular gyri
Lateral sulcus
Superior temporal gyrus and sulcus
Occipital lobe

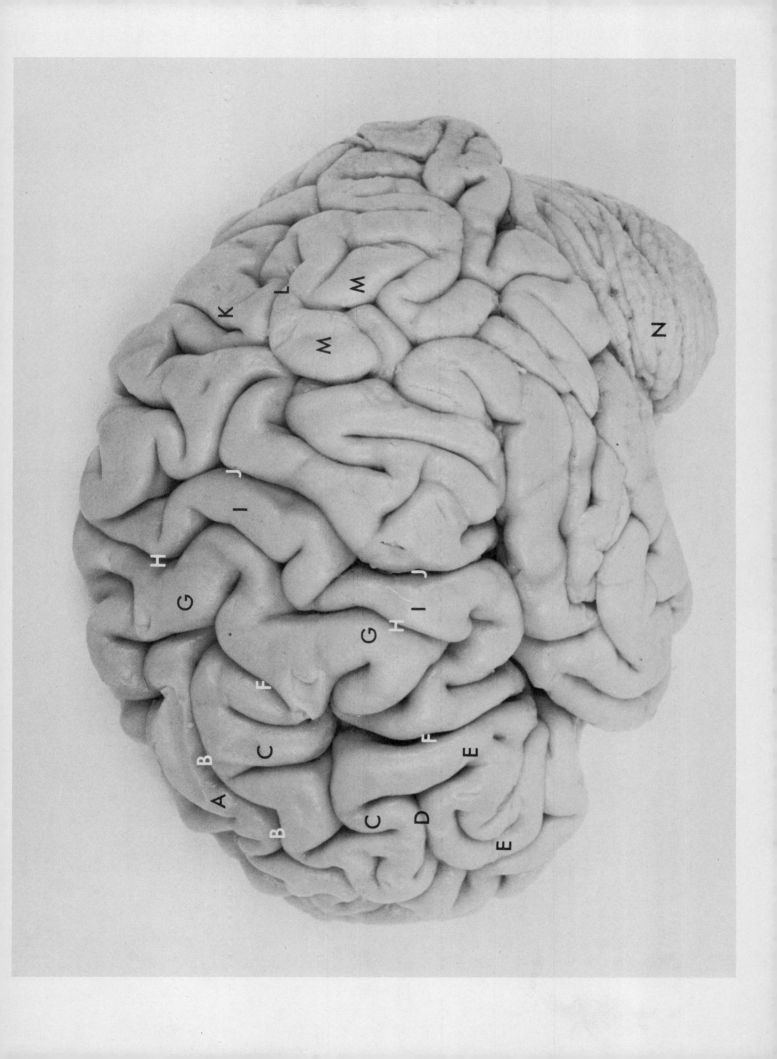

Figure 12. Medial View of the Brain, Arachnoid and Pia Mater Removed. Midsagittal Section (×1.5)

A. Straight gyrus (gyrus rectus)
B. Paraterminal gyrus
C. Subcallosal area
D. Cingulate gyrus
E. Cingulate sulcus (and its marginal ramus)
F. Paracentral lobule
G. Central sulcus
H. Precuneus
I. Parietooccipital sulcus
J. Calcarine sulcus
K. Splenium of corpus callosum
L. Trunk of corpus callosum
M. Genu of corpus callosum
N. Rostrum of corpus callosum
O. Septum pellucidum
P. Body of fornix
Q. Choroid plexus of lateral ventricle
R. Pineal body
S. Interthalamic adhesion
T. Anterior commissure
U. Cerebral aqueduct
V. Superior medullary velum
W. Fourth ventricle

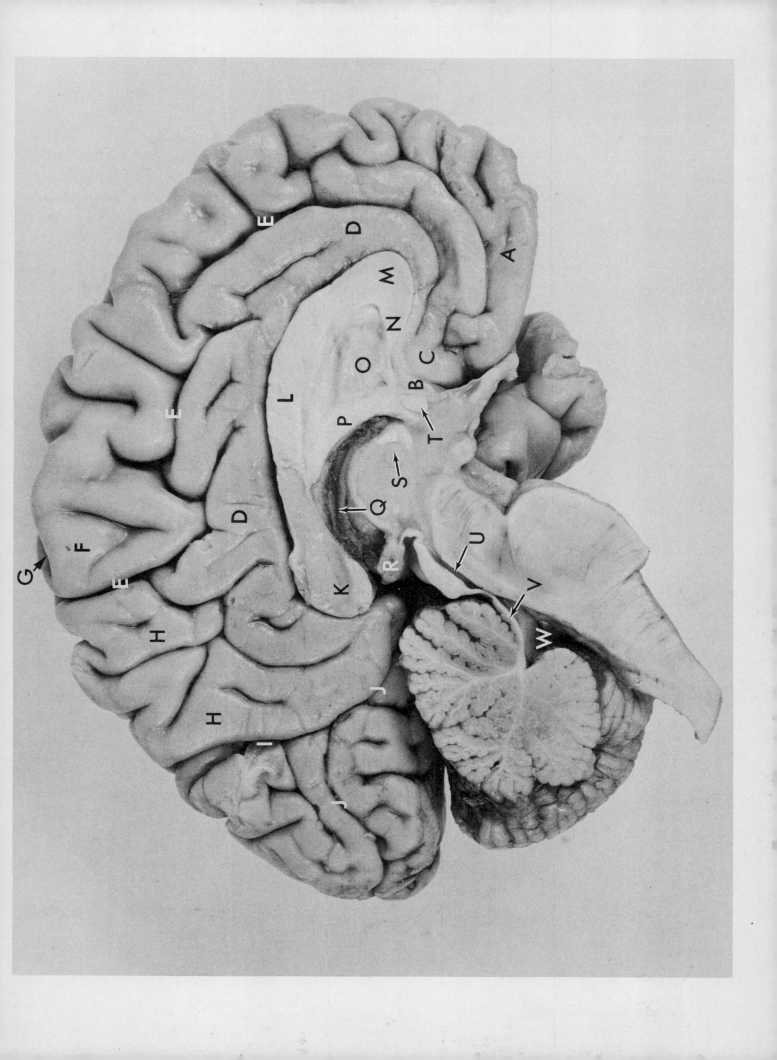

Figure 13. Medial View of the Brain, Arachnoid and Pia Mater Removed. Midsagittal Section (×1.5)

A. Superior frontal gyrus
B. Cingulate sulcus
C. Cingulate gyrus
D. Isthmus of cingulate gyrus
E. Parietooccipital sulcus
F. Cuneus
G. Calcarine sulcus
H. Lingual gyrus
I. Interventricular foramen
J. Thalamus
K. Hypothalamic sulcus (position of)
L. Hypothalamus
M. Optic recess of third ventricle
N. Optic chiasma
O. Infundibulum and infundibular recess of third ventricle
P. Tuber cinereum
Q. Mammillary body
R. Posterior commissure
S. Superior colliculus
T. Inferior colliculus
U. Cerebral peduncle of midbrain
V. Pons
W. Medulla
X. Cerebellum (vermis)
Y. Cerebellum (hemisphere)

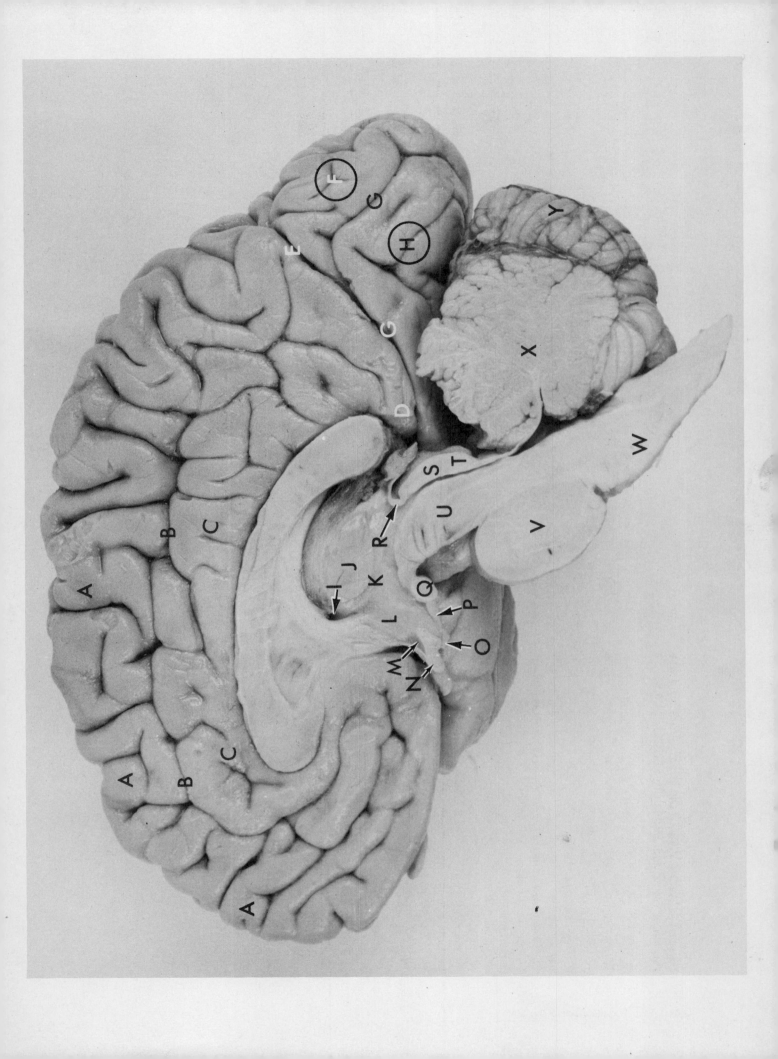

HORIZONTAL SECTIONS OF THE BRAIN
(WITH CT SCAN CORRELATION)

Figure 14. Photograph of the Brain Indicating the Approximate Level and Plane of Figures 15–22 (LeMasurier Modification of the Mulligan Stain)

The next eight sections are cut to approximate, in level and plane, the cuts made by the new neuroradiological technique known as computerized tomography, or CT scanning. These cuts are made at an angle of approximately 15 degrees to the orbitomeatal line and are illustrated on the photograph on the next page.

It is hoped that the student will be able to identify, on the normal and abnormal CT scans, many of the anatomical structures that are labeled on the brain sections. In addition, the student should attempt to correlate the position of other important structures, not visible on CT scan, by using the relationships that are clearly visible on the brain sections.

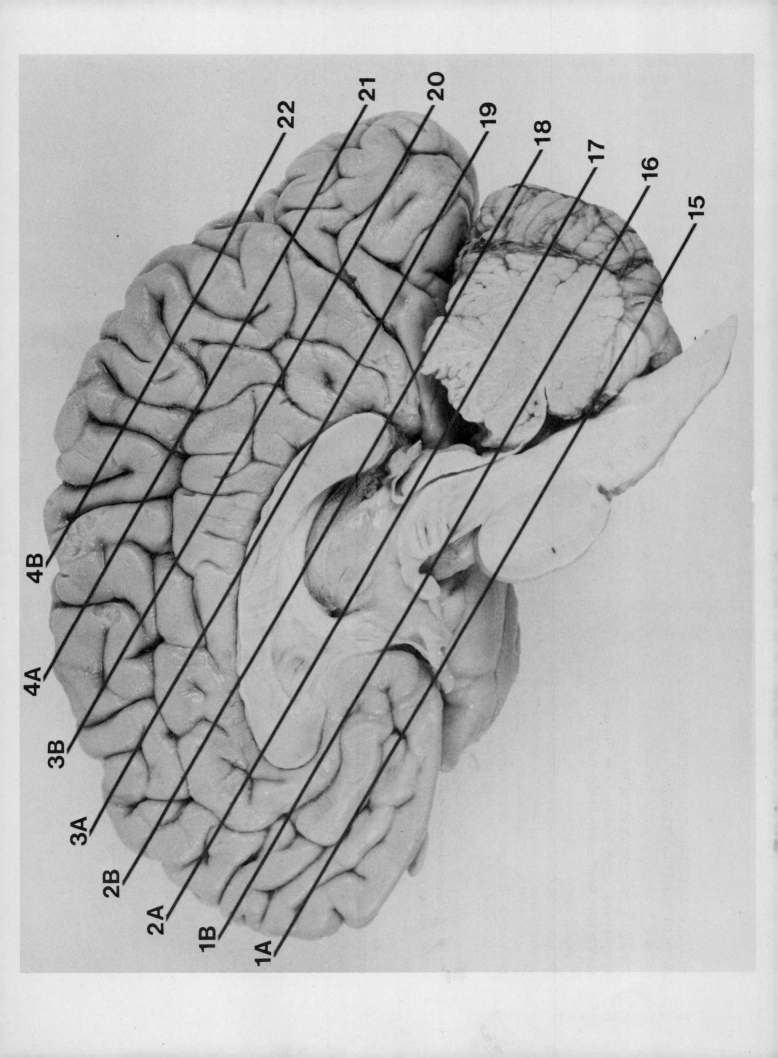

Figure 15. Angled Horizontal Section of the Brain Passing Through the Cerebellum, Pons, Infundibulum, and Optic Chiasma (Approximately Equivalent to the 1A Level of the CT Scan) (×1.25)

A. Longitudinal cerebral fissure
B. Frontal lobe
C. Lateral sulcus
D. Optic chiasma (surrounded by the *chiasmatic cistern*)
E. Infundibulum
F. Middle cerebral artery
G. Temporal lobe
H. Amygdaloid body
 I. Inferior horn of lateral ventricle
J. Hippocampus
K. Position of interpeduncular cistern or sella turcica (depending on level of the section)
L. Prepontine cistern
M. Pons (just above level of trigeminal nerves)
N. Fourth ventricle
O. Cerebellar vermis
P. Cerebellar hemisphere
Q. Cerebellomedullary cistern (cisterna magna)
R. Position of petrous part of temporal bone (on CT scan)

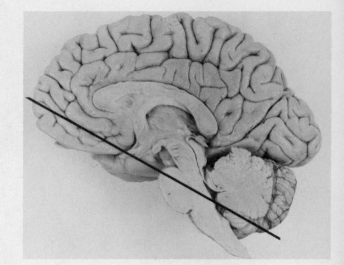

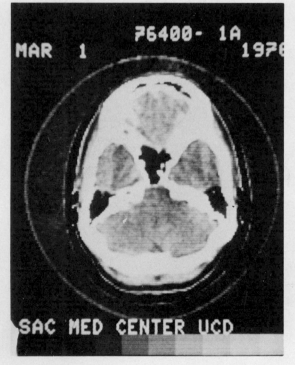

Normal CT scan.

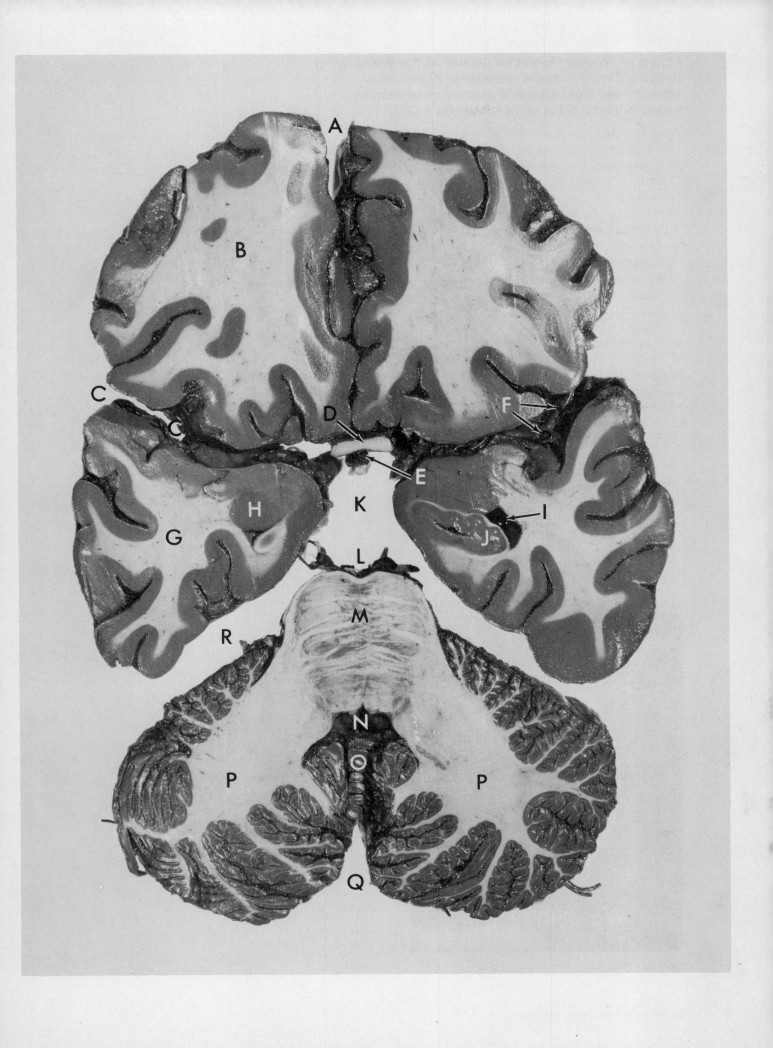

Figure 16. Angled Horizontal Section of the Brain Passing Through the Cerebellum, Midbrain, Mammillary Bodies, and Lamina Terminalis (Approximately Equivalent to the 1B Level of the CT Scan) (×1.25)

A. Frontal lobe
B. Rostrum of corpus callosum
C. Anterior cerebral arteries (running in the *longitudinal cerebral fissure*)
D. Lamina terminalis (*cistern of the lamina terminalis* is just anterior to this structure)
E. Third ventricle (inferior part)
F. Hypothalamus
G. Column of fornix (entering mammillary body)
H. Mammillary body
I. Interpeduncular cistern
J. Optic tract
K. Ambient cistern
L. Midbrain
M. Fourth ventricle
N. Cerebellar vermis
O. Cerebellar hemisphere
P. Dentate nucleus of cerebellum
Q. Dentatorubrothalamic tract (leaving the dentate nucleus and ascending, via the *superior cerebellar peduncle*, to the midbrain)
R. Temporal lobe
S. Inferior horn of lateral ventricle
T. Hippocampus
U. Putamen of lentiform nucleus
V. Head of caudate nucleus
W. Anterior limb of internal capsule
X. Tip of anterior horn of lateral ventricle
Y. Lateral sulcus (with branches of middle cerebral artery in it)

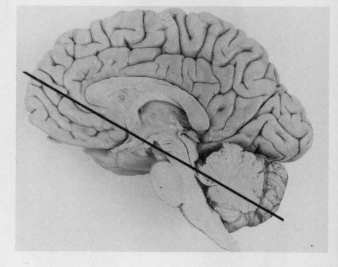

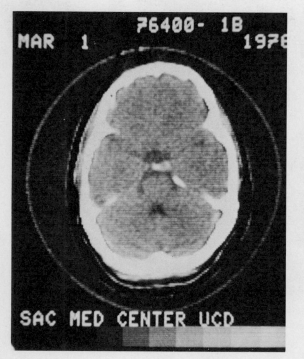

Normal CT scan.

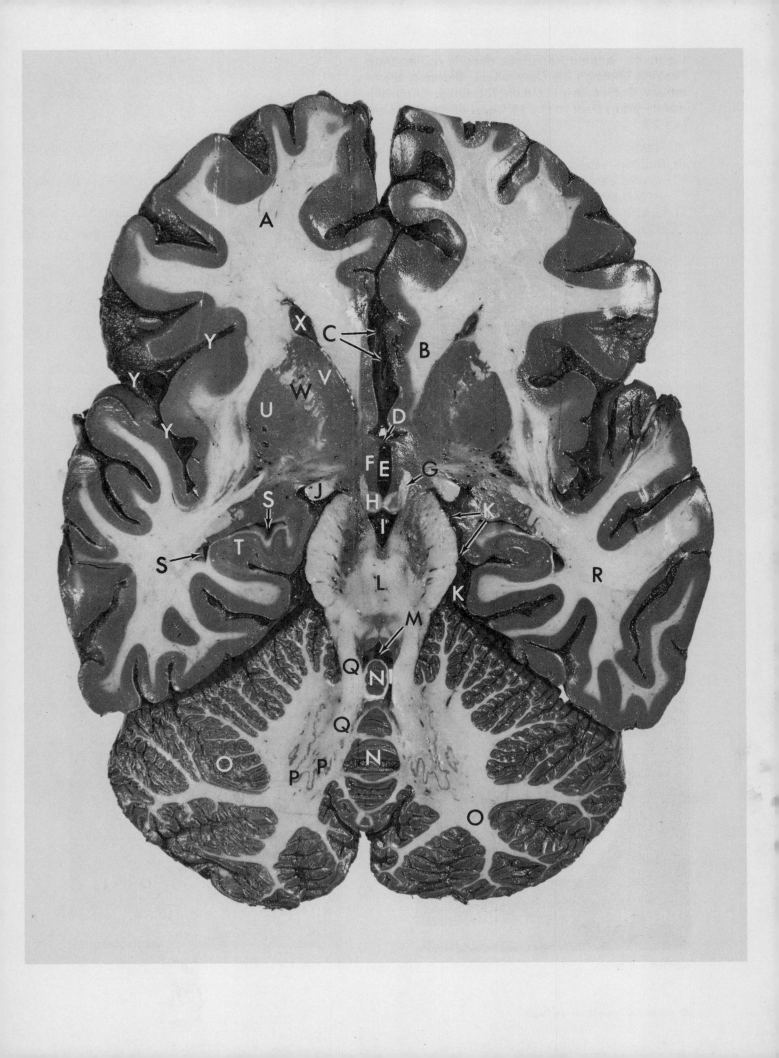

Figure 17. Angled Horizontal Section of the Brain Passing Through the Cerebellum, Superior Colliculi, Third Ventricle, Body of the Fornix, and Genu of the Corpus Callosum (Approximately Equivalent to the 2A Level of the CT Scan) (×1.25)

A. Frontal lobe
B. Cingulate gyrus
C. Anterior cerebral arteries (pericallosal branches)
D. Genu of corpus callosum
E. Anterior horn of lateral ventricle
F. Septum pellucidum
G. Body of fornix
H. Arrow passing through the interventricular foramen (from lateral ventricle to third ventricle)
I. Head of caudate nucleus
J. Anterior limb of internal capsule
K. Genu of internal capsule
L. Posterior limb of internal capsule
M. Putamen of lentiform nucleus
N. Globus pallidus of lentiform nucleus
O. Thalamus
P. Medial geniculate body of thalamus
Q. Lateral geniculate body of thalamus
R. Interthalamic adhesion
S. Third ventricle
T. Superior colliculus (lower tip)
U. Superior (or quadrigeminal) cistern
V. Cerebellum
W. Temporal lobe

X. Tail of caudate nucleus (in roof of *inferior horn of lateral ventricle*)
Y. Hippocampus and its fimbria (in floor of *inferior horn of lateral ventricle*)
Z. From the putamen lateralward: external capsule (white), claustrum (gray), extreme capsule (white), and insula (gray cortex)

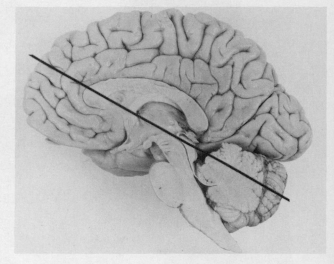

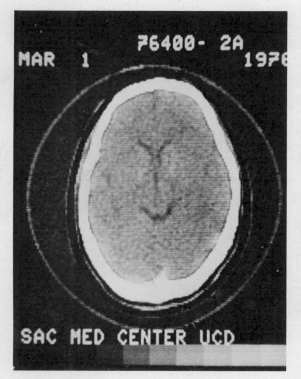

Normal CT scan.

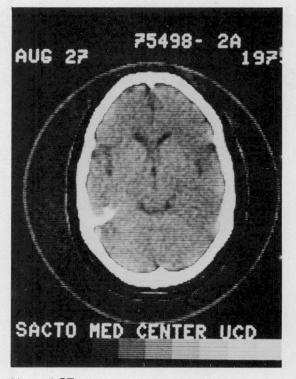

Normal CT scan.

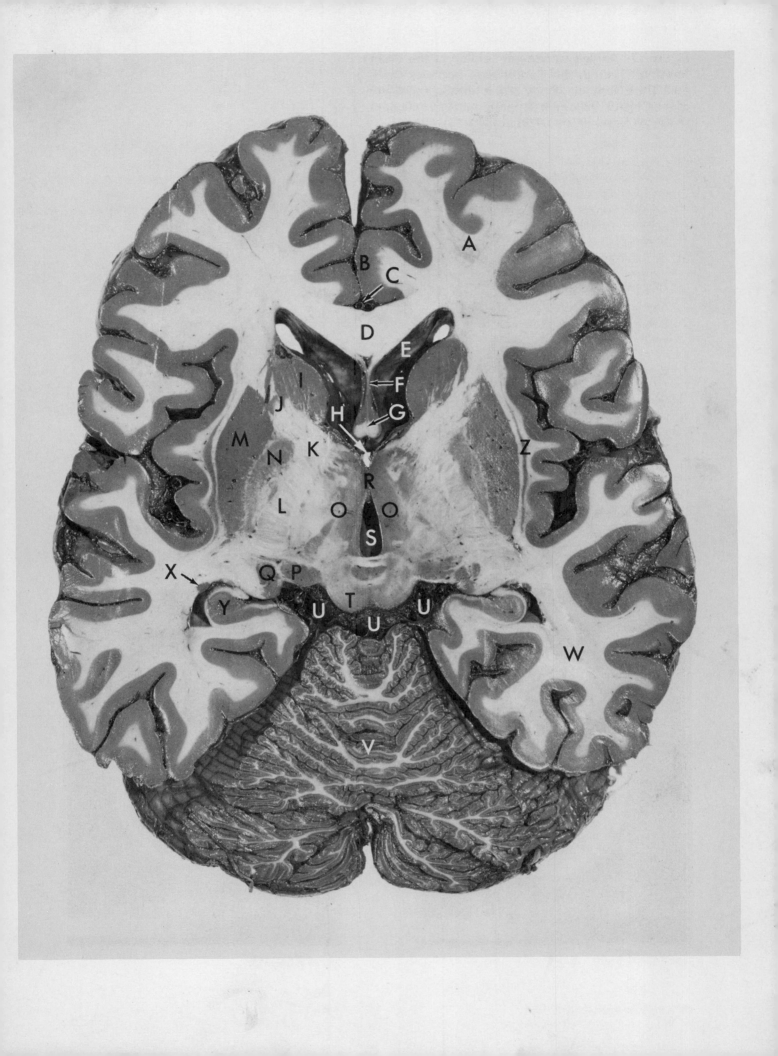

Figure 18. Angled Horizontal Section of the Brain Passing Through the Splenium of the Corpus Callosum, Crura of the Fornix, Septum Pellucidum, and Trunk of the Corpus Callosum (Approximately Equivalent to the 2B Level of the CT Scan) (×1.25)

A. Frontal lobe
B. Trunk of corpus callosum
C. Anterior horn of lateral ventricle
D. Septum pellucidum
E. Choroid plexus of lateral ventricle
F. Thalamostriate vein
G. Head of caudate nucleus
H. Thalamus
 I. Crus of fornix (two places)
J. Anterior extension of superior cistern within the transverse cerebral fissure (contains the two *internal cerebral veins*, which are difficult to see here)
K. Splenium of corpus callosum
L. Great cerebral vein (within superior cistern) (the calcified *pineal body* is frequently seen in CT scans at this location)
M. Superior surface of cerebellum
N. Occipital lobe
O. Calcarine sulcus
P. Choroid plexus within inferior horn of lateral ventricle (frequently seen in CT scans at this location)
Q. Tail of caudate nucleus
R. Temporal lobe
S. Corona radiata (just above internal capsule)
T. Lateral sulcus (with several branches of middle cerebral artery within it)

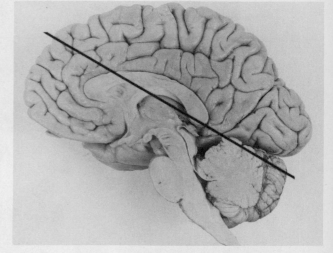

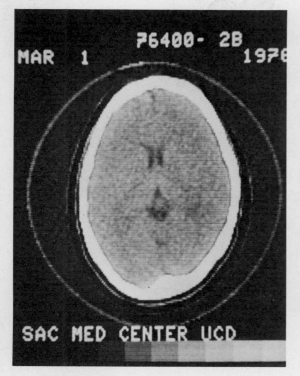

Normal CT scan.

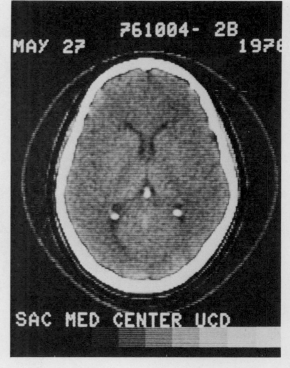

Normal CT scan.

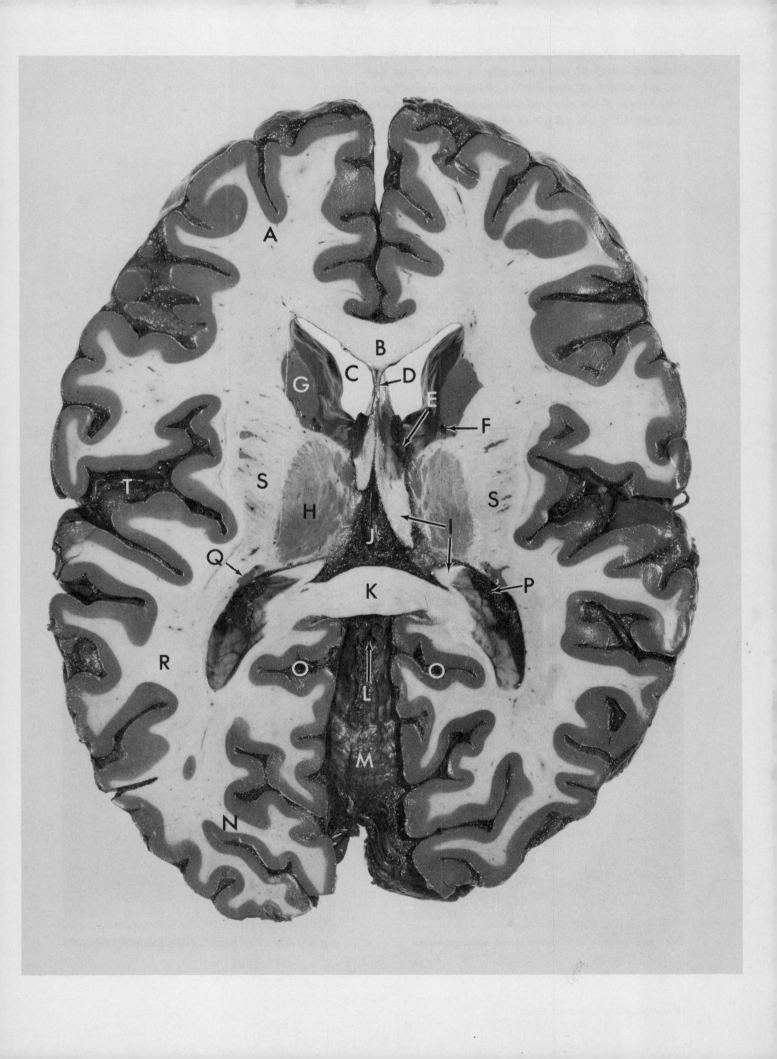

Figure 19. Angled Horizontal Section of the Cerebrum Passing Through the Collateral Trigone and Central Part of the Lateral Ventricles and the Top of the Trunk of the Corpus Callosum (Approximately Equivalent to the 3A Level of the CT Scan) (×1.25)

A. Longitudinal cerebral fissure
B. Frontal lobe
C. Top of trunk of corpus callosum
D. Central part of lateral ventricle
E. Choroid plexus (frequently seen in CT scans at this location)
F. Collateral trigone of lateral ventricle
G. Posterior forceps of corpus callosum
H. Calcarine sulcus
 I. Occipital lobe
J. Temporal lobe
K. Superior temporal sulcus
L. Lateral sulcus
M. Parietal lobe
N. Central sulcus
O. Precentral sulcus
P. Corona radiata

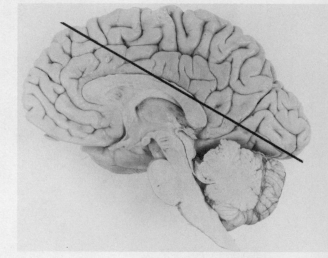

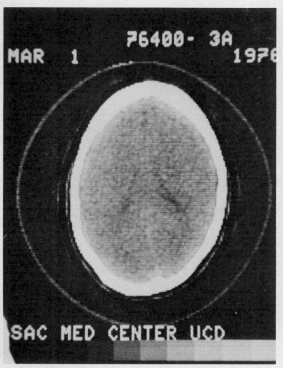

Normal CT scan.

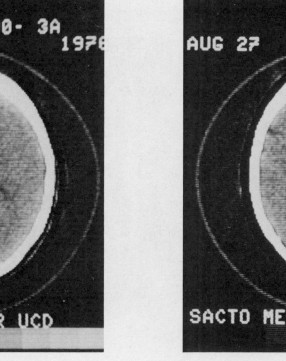

Normal CT scan showing the posterior horn of the lateral ventricle.

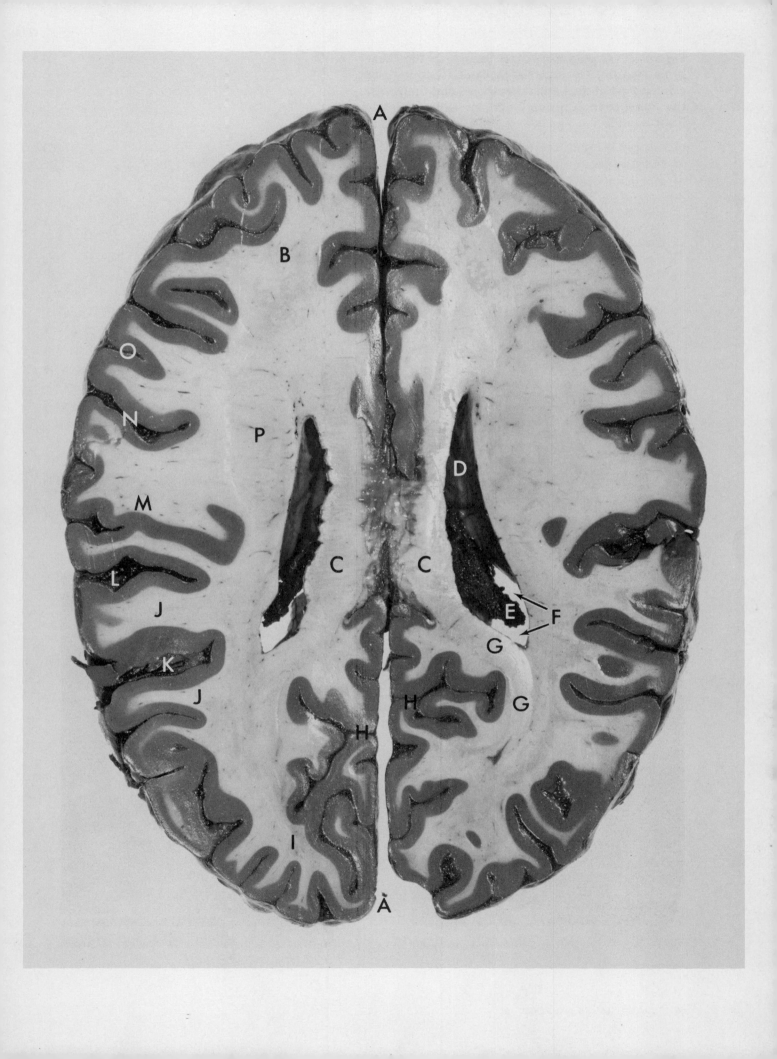

Figure 20. Angled Horizontal Section of the Cerebrum Passing Through the Occipital, Parietal, and Frontal Lobes (Approximately Equivalent to the 3B Level of the CT Scan) (×1.25)

A. Longitudinal cerebral fissure
B. Frontal lobe
C. Precentral sulcus
D. Precentral gyrus
E. Central sulcus
F. Postcentral gyrus
G. Postcentral sulcus
H. Parietal lobe
I. Parietooccipital sulcus
J. Occipital lobe

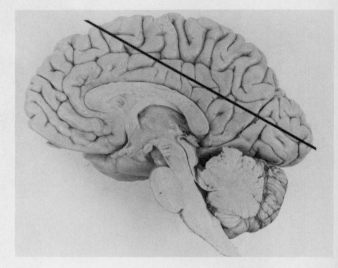

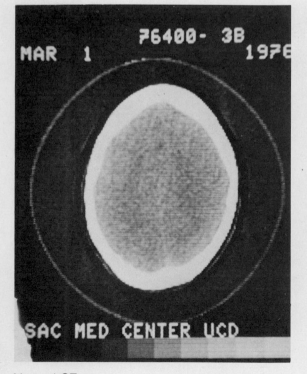

Normal CT scan.

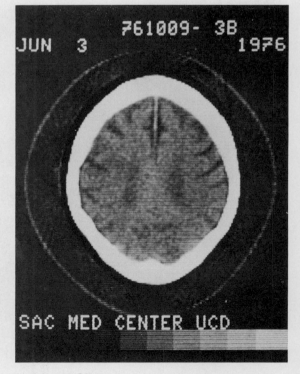

Abnormal CT scan showing cortical atrophy.

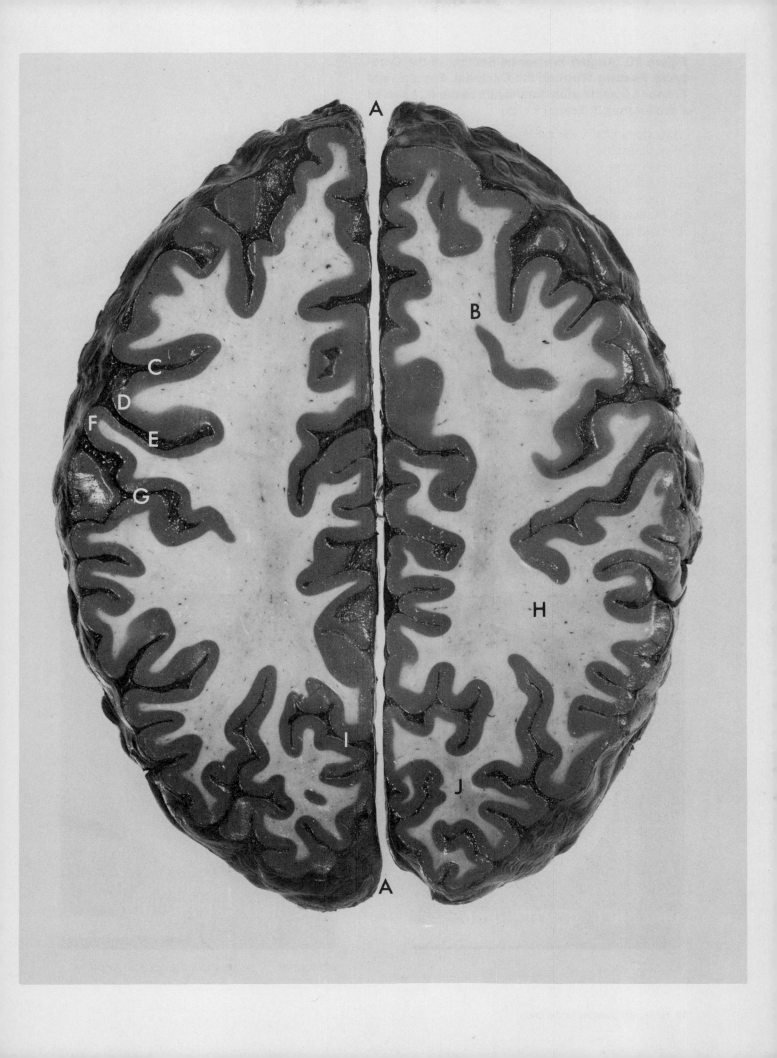

Figure 21. Angled Horizontal Section of the Cerebrum Passing Through the Frontal and Parietal Lobes (Approximately Equivalent to the 4A Level of the CT Scan) (×1.5)

A. Longitudinal cerebral fissure (note the calcified *falx cerebri* within this fissure on the CT scan with cortical atrophy)
B. Frontal lobe
C. Precentral sulcus
D. Precentral gyrus
E. Central sulcus (note the widening of the sulci on the abnormal CT scan with cortical atrophy)
F. Postcentral gyrus
G. Postcentral sulcus
H. Parietal lobe
I. Top of parietooccipital sulcus

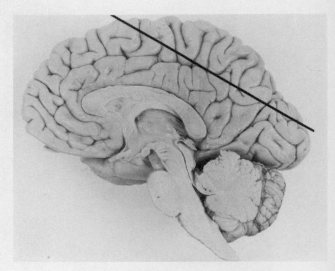

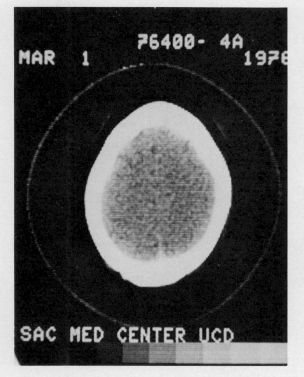

Normal CT scan.

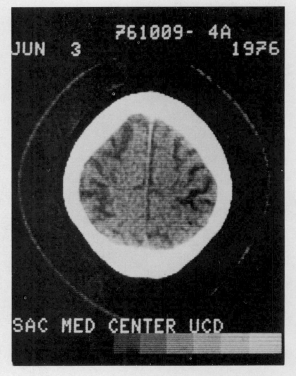

Abnormal CT scan showing cortical atrophy.

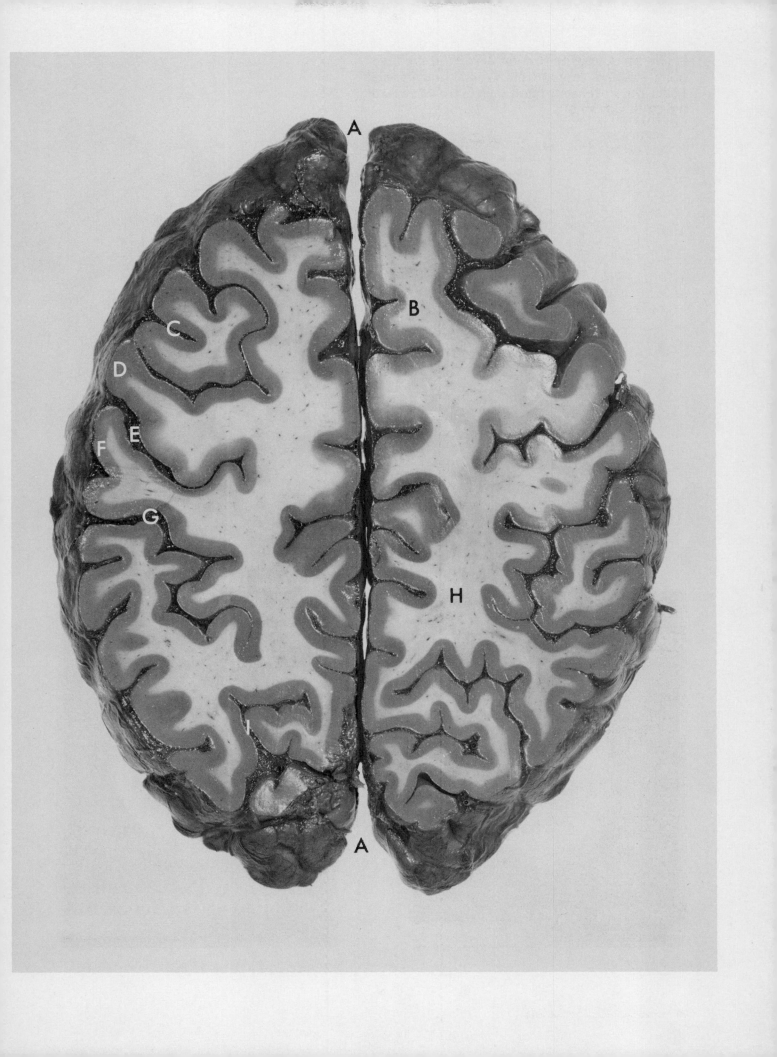

Figure 22. Angled Horizontal Section of the Cerebrum Passing Through the Posterior Frontal Lobe and the Superior Aspect of the Parietal Lobe (Approximately Equivalent to the 4B Level of the CT Scan) (×2)

A. Longitudinal cerebral fissure (note calcified *falx cerebri* within this fissure on abnormal CT scan)
B. Frontal lobe
C. Precentral sulcus
D. Precentral gyrus
E. Central sulcus (note the cortical atrophy causing widening of the sulci on the abnormal CT scan)
F. Postcentral gyrus
G. Postcentral sulcus
H. Parietal lobe

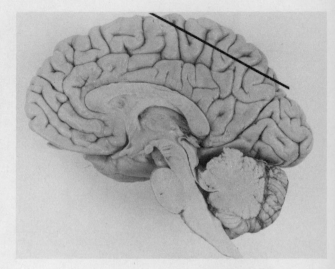

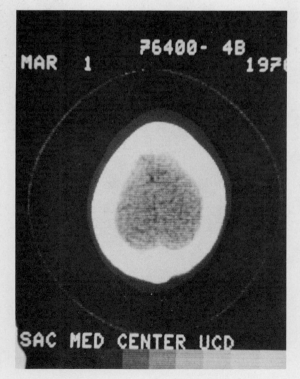

Normal CT scan.

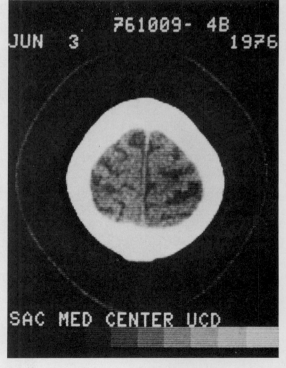

Abnormal CT scan showing cortical atrophy.

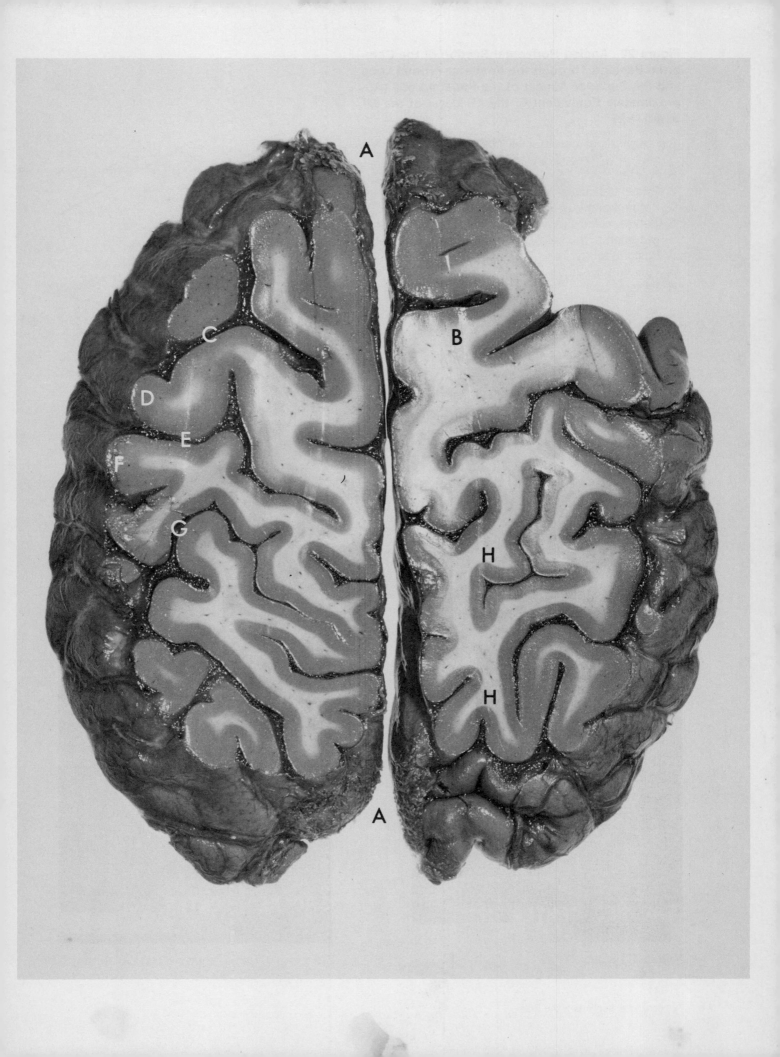

FRONTAL SECTIONS OF THE CEREBRUM AND DIENCEPHALON AND TRANSVERSE SECTIONS OF THE BRAINSTEM

Figure 23. Photograph of the Brain Indicating the Approximate Level and Plane of Figures 24–33 (LeMasurier Modification of the Mulligan Stain)

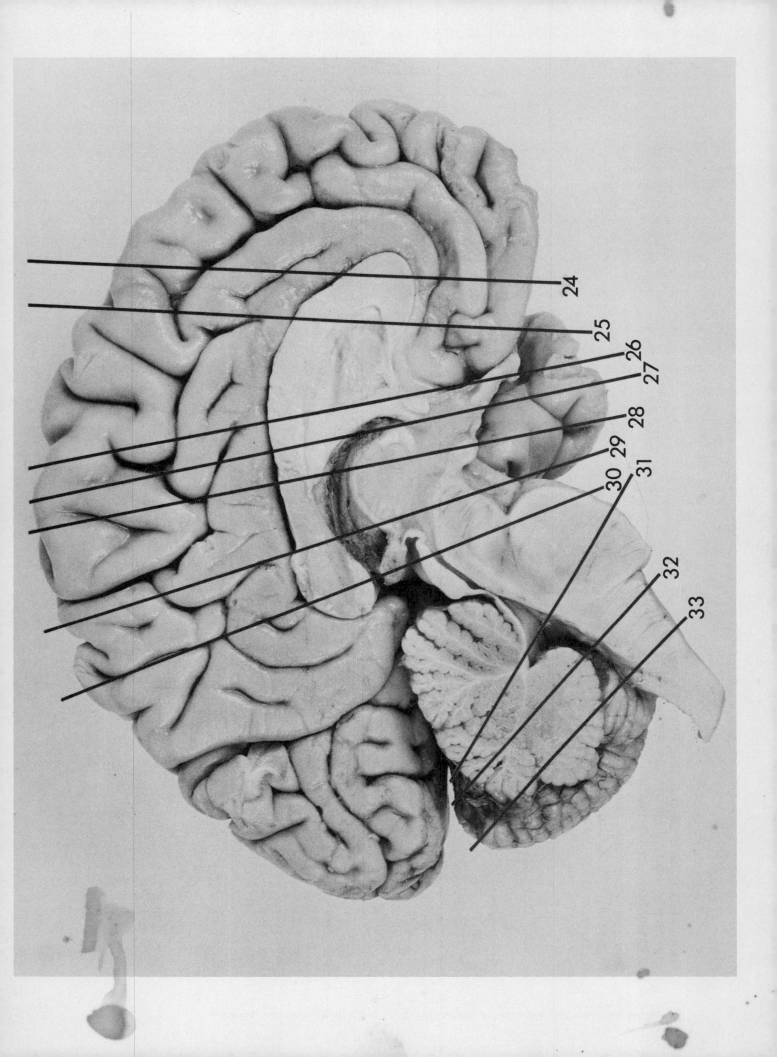

24

25

26

27

28

29

30

31

32

33

Figure 24. Frontal Section of the Cerebral Hemispheres Passing Through the Genu of the Corpus Callosum (×2)

A. Cerebral cortex (gray matter)
B. Centrum semiovale (white matter)
C. Superior frontal gyrus
D. Superior frontal sulcus
E. Middle frontal gyrus
F. Inferior frontal sulcus
G. Inferior frontal gyrus
H. Orbital gyri
I. Orbital sulci
J. Olfactory sulcus
K. Straight gyrus (gyrus rectus)
L. Longitudinal cerebral fissure
M. Cingulate sulcus
N. Cingulate gyrus
O. Genu of corpus callosum
P. Anterior horn of right lateral ventricle
Q. Head of caudate nucleus
R. Anterior cerebral arteries (two places)
S. Arachnoid (spans the sulcus)
T. Pia mater (dips into the sulcus)

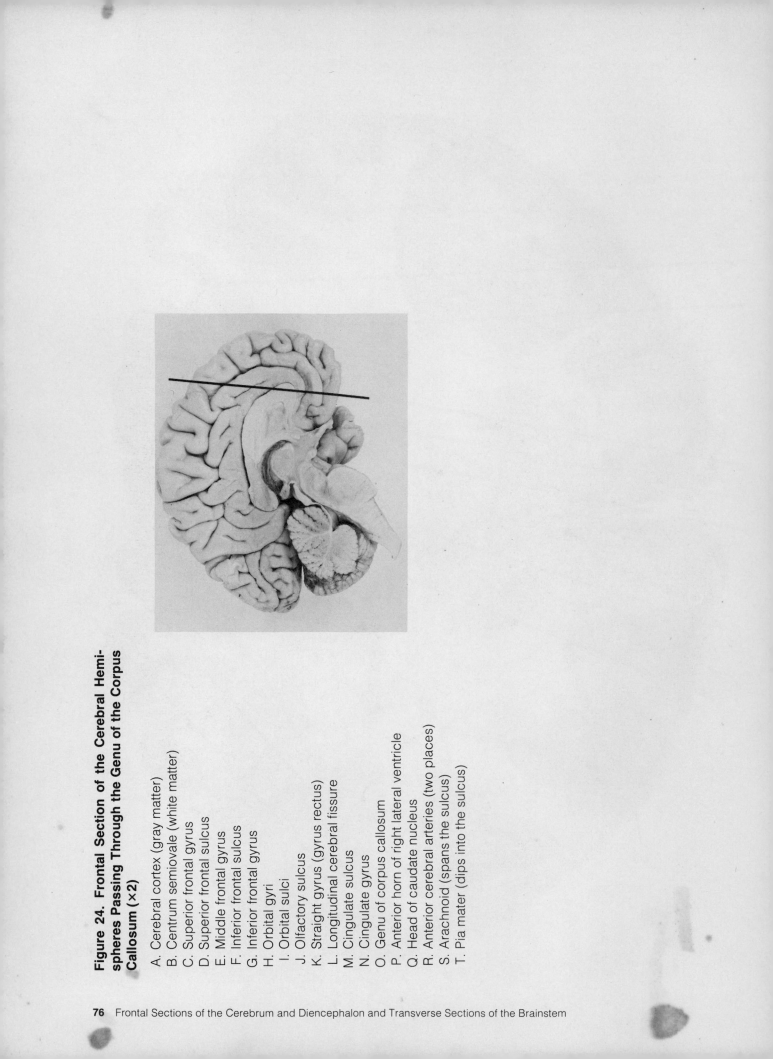

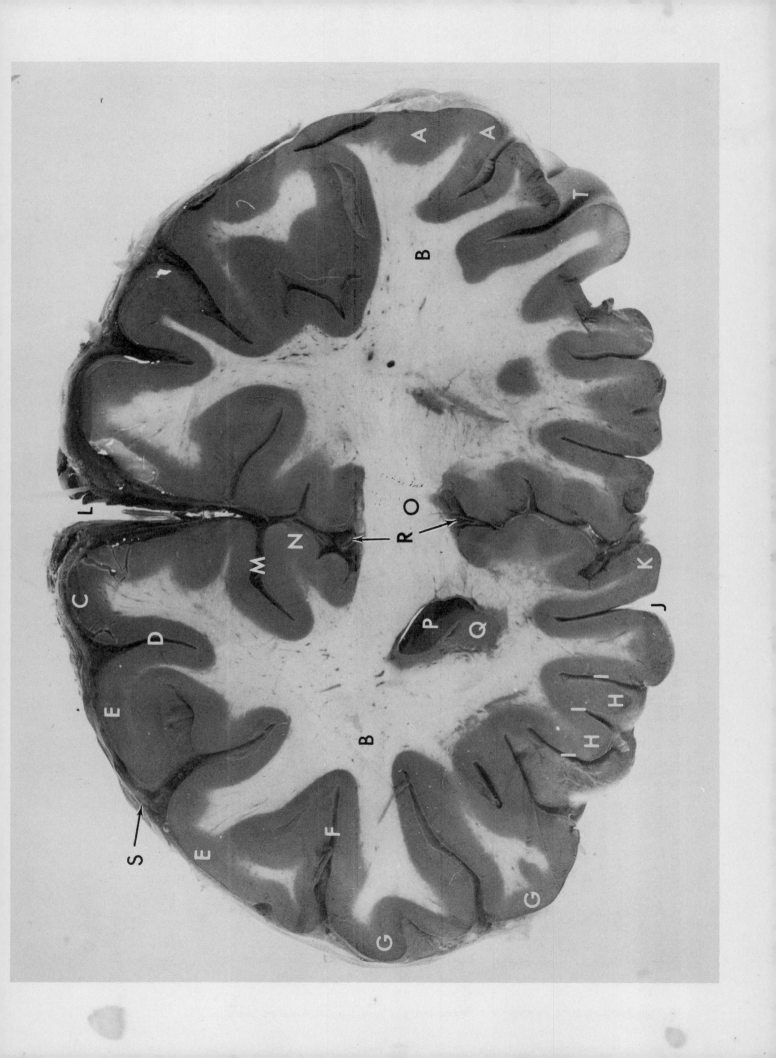

Figure 25. Frontal Section of the Cerebral Hemispheres Passing Through the Rostrum of the Corpus Callosum (×1.5)

A. Cingulate sulcus
B. Cingulate gyrus
C. Trunk of corpus callosum
D. Septum pellucidum
E. Rostrum of corpus callosum
F. Olfactory tract (in olfactory sulcus)
G. Anterior horn of lateral ventricle
H. Head of caudate nucleus
I. Putamen (of lentiform nucleus)
J. External capsule
K. Claustrum
L. Extreme capsule
M. Middle cerebral artery (in lateral sulcus)
N. Temporal lobe
O. Arachnoid (spans the sulci)

Can you locate:

Longitudinal cerebral fissure
Anterior cerebral arteries

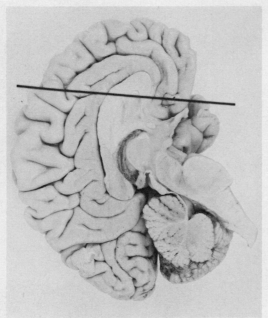

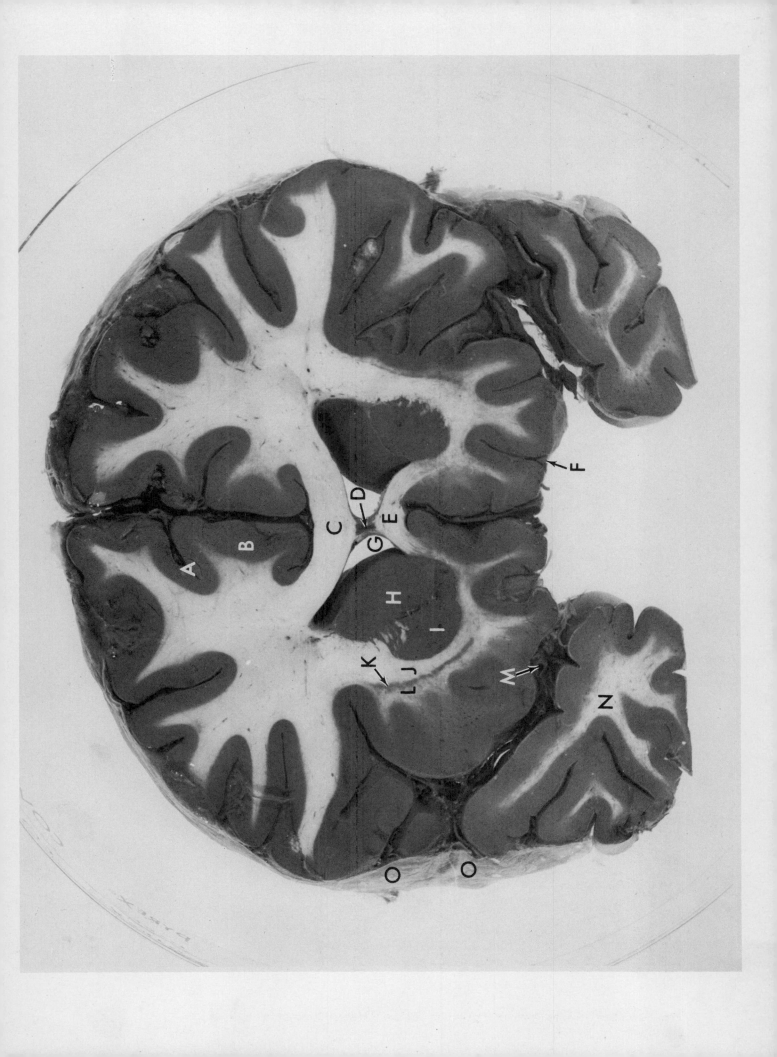

Figure 26. Frontal Section of the Cerebral Hemispheres Passing Through the Optic Chiasma (×1.5)

A. Superior frontal gyrus (bounded inferiorly by *superior frontal sulcus*)
B. Middle frontal gyrus
C. Inferior frontal gyrus (bounded superiorly by *inferior frontal sulcus*)
D. Lateral sulcus
E. Superior temporal gyrus (bounded by *superior temporal sulcus* inferiorly)
F. Middle temporal gyrus (bounded by *middle temporal sulcus* inferiorly)
G. Inferior temporal gyrus
H. Inferior temporal sulcus
I. Occipitotemporal gyrus
J. Uncus (bounded laterally by *collateral sulcus*)
K. Trunk of corpus callosum
L. Septum pellucidum (separating the anterior horns of *left* and *right lateral ventricles*)
M. Paraterminal gyrus
N. Optic chiasma
O. Head of caudate nucleus
P. Corona radiata
Q. Anterior limb of internal capsule
R. Putamen of lentiform nucleus
S. External capsule

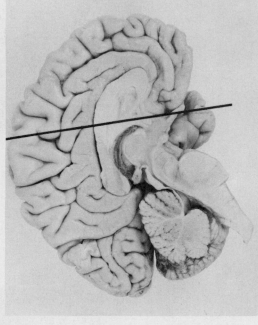

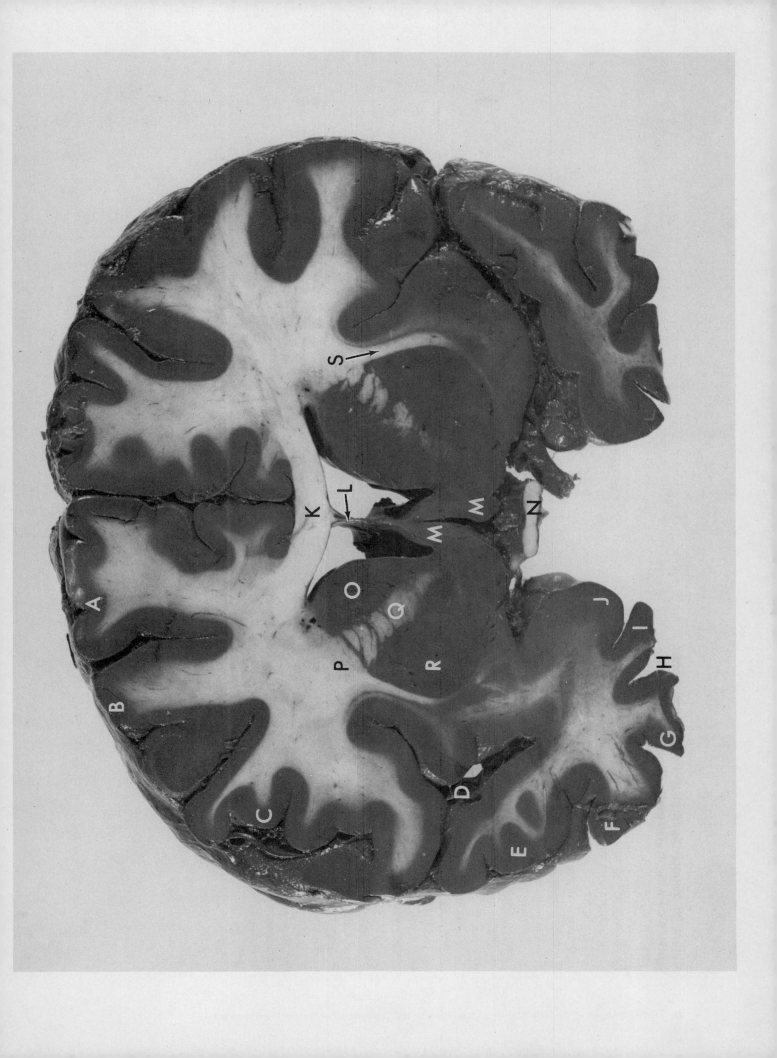

Figure 27. Frontal Section of the Cerebral Hemispheres Passing Through the Infundibulum (×1.5)

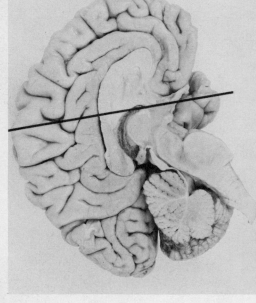

A. Choroid plexus of lateral ventricle
B. Body of fornix
C. Interventricular foramen
D. Third ventricle (locate the hypothalamic sulcus and the choroid plexus)
E. Column of fornix
F. Hypothalamus
G. Infundibulum (note that the cavity of the third ventricle extends into the infundibulum as the infundibular recess)
H. Optic tract
I. Anterior end of thalamus
J. Body of caudate nucleus
K. Internal capsule (near *genu*)
L. Corona radiata
M. Globus pallidus of lentiform nucleus
N. Putamen of lentiform nucleus
O. Insula
P. Lateral sulcus (with middle cerebral artery in it)
Q. Superior temporal gyrus (bounded inferiorly by *superior temporal sulcus*)
R. Middle temporal gyrus (bounded inferiorly by *middle temporal sulcus*)
S. Inferior temporal gyrus
T. Occipitotemporal gyrus (bounded laterally by *inferior temporal sulcus*)
U. Uncus (bounded laterally by *collateral sulcus*)
V. Amygdaloid body
W. Anterior commissure
X. Ansa lenticularis

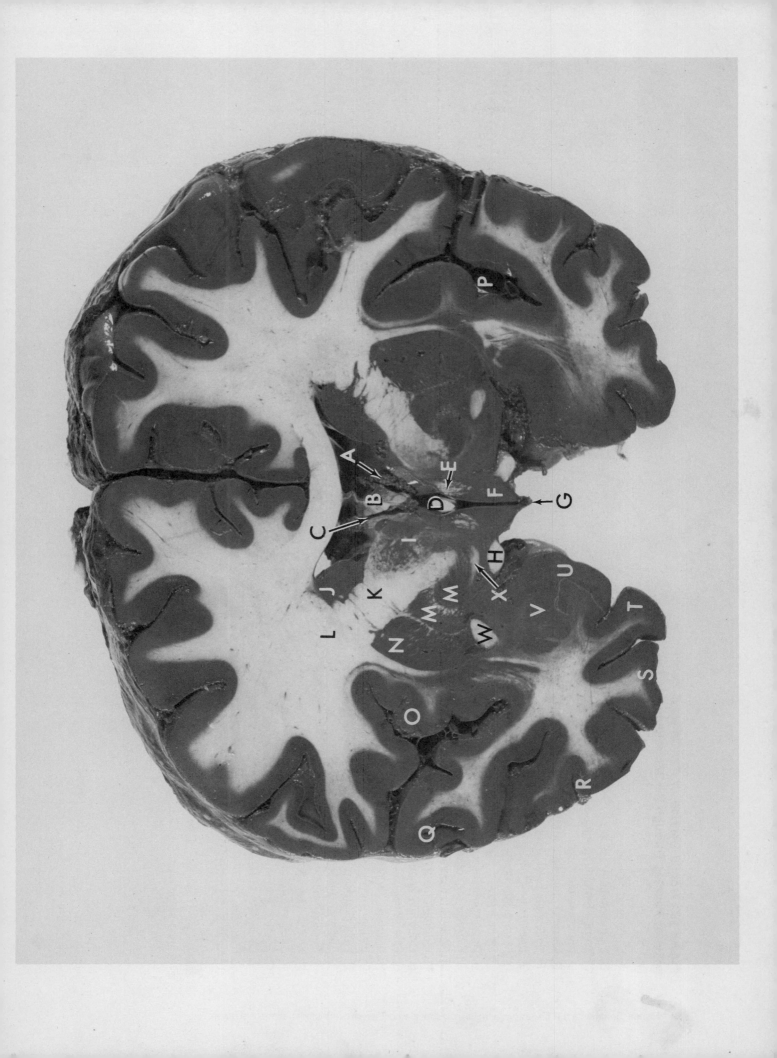

Figure 28. Frontal Section of the Cerebral Hemispheres Passing Through the Mammillary Bodies (×1.5)

A. Central part of lateral ventricle
B. Lateral thalamic nuclei
C. Medial thalamic nuclei
D. Interthalamic adhesion
E. Mammillothalamic tract
F. Lenticular fasciculus
G. Subthalamic nucleus
H. Mammillary body
I. Optic tract
J. Posterior limb of internal capsule
K. Crus cerebri of cerebral peduncle
L. Globus pallidus of lentiform nucleus
M. Putamen of lentiform nucleus
N. External capsule
O. Claustrum
P. Extreme capsule
Q. Insula
R. Amygdaloid body
S. Inferior horn of lateral ventricle
T. Parahippocampal gyrus
U. Occipitotemporal gyrus
V. Inferior temporal gyrus

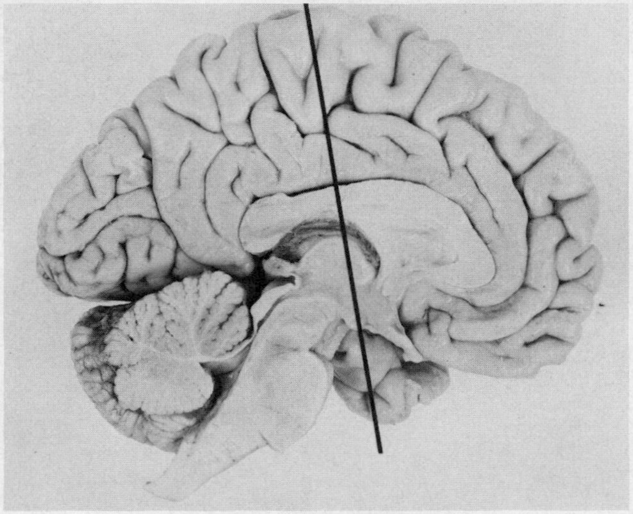

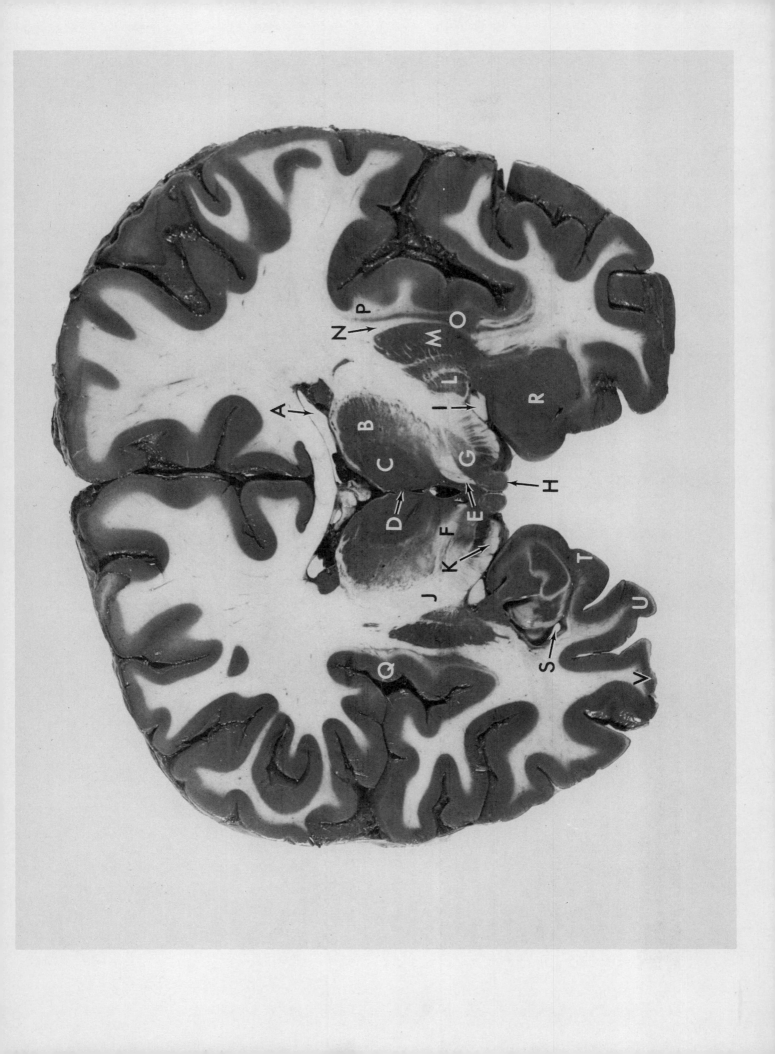

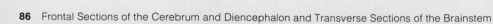

Figure 29. Frontal Section of the Cerebral Hemispheres Passing Through the Rostral End of the Red Nucleus (×1.5)

A. Caudate nucleus (near the body-tail juncture)
B. Choroid plexus of lateral ventricle
C. Crus of fornix
D. Third ventricle
E. Medial thalamic nuclei
F. Lateral thalamic nuclei
G. Posterior end of lentiform nucleus (mostly putamen)
H. Posterior limb of internal capsule
I. Crus cerebri of cerebral peduncle
J. Substantia nigra of cerebral peduncle
K. Red nucleus
L. Optic tract
M. Inferior horn of lateral ventricle
N. Hippocampus
O. Parahippocampal gyrus
P. Collateral sulcus
Q. Occipitotemporal gyrus
R. Interpeduncular fossa

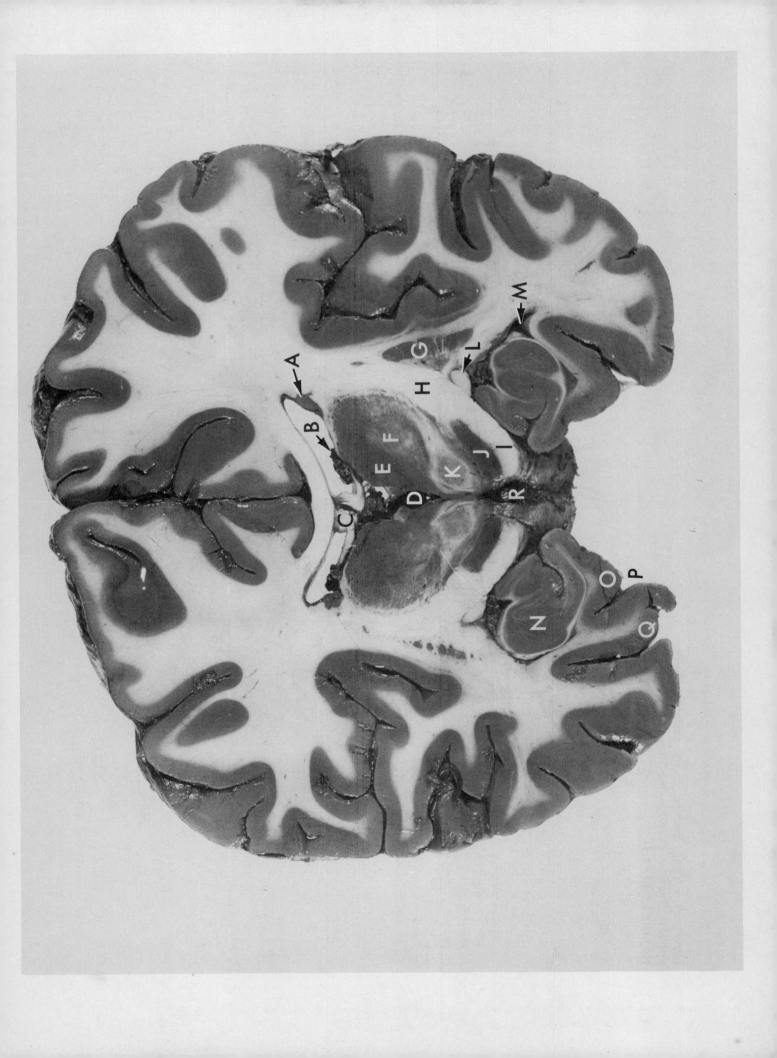

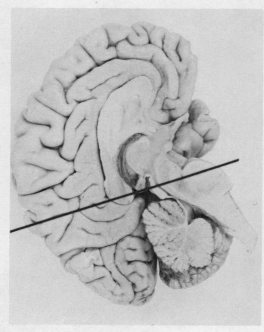

Figure 30. Frontal Section of the Cerebral Hemispheres Passing Through the Geniculate Bodies of the Thalamus (×1.5)

A. Cingulate gyrus (bounded above by *cingulate sulcus*)
B. Splenium of corpus callosum
C. Choroid plexus of central part of lateral ventricle
D. Crus of fornix
E. Thalamus (pulvinar)
F. Lateral geniculate body of thalamus
G. Medial geniculate body of thalamus
H. Pretectal area
I. Central gray substance of midbrain (hole in the middle of this is the *cerebral aqueduct*)
J. Medial longitudinal fasciculus
K. Superior cerebellar peduncle (soon to enter the red nucleus rostrally)
L. Substantia nigra of cerebral peduncle
M. Crus cerebri of cerebral peduncle
N. Pons
O. Tail of caudate nucleus (two places)
P. Inferior horn of lateral ventricle
Q. Hippocampus
R. Fimbria of hippocampus (two places)
S. Parahippocampal gyrus

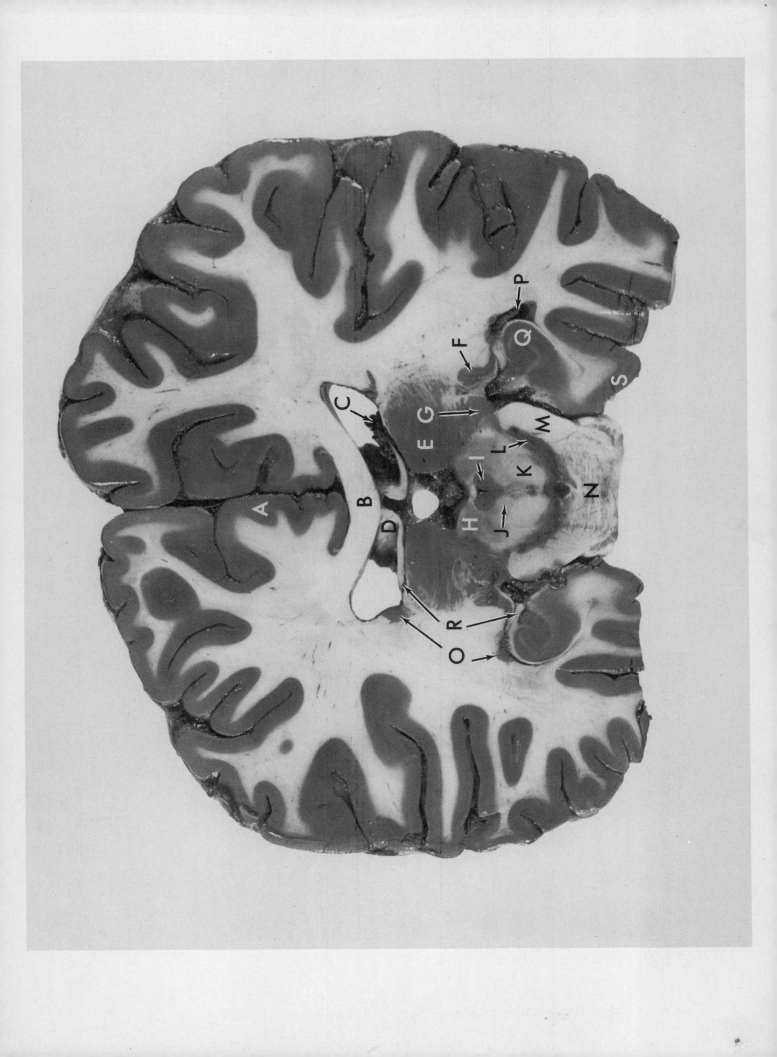

Figure 31. Transverse Section of the Metencephalon Passing Through the Midpons (or Slightly Below) (×3)

A. Cerebellar hemisphere
B. Vermis of cerebellum
C. Flocculus of cerebellum
D. Fourth ventricle
E. Superior cerebellar peduncle
F. Inferior cerebellar peduncle
G. Middle cerebellar peduncle
H. Tegmentum, or dorsal, part of pons
I. Basal, or ventral, part of pons
J. Basilar artery (lying in the *basilar sulcus* of the pons)

Can you locate:

Trapezoid body
Medial lemniscus
Lateral lemniscus
Superior olivary nucleus
Pontine nuclei
Pyramidal tract (corticospinal and corticonuclear fibers)

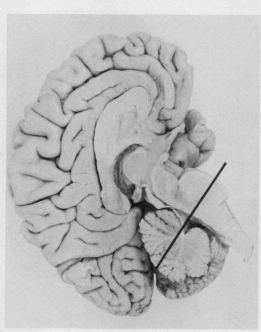

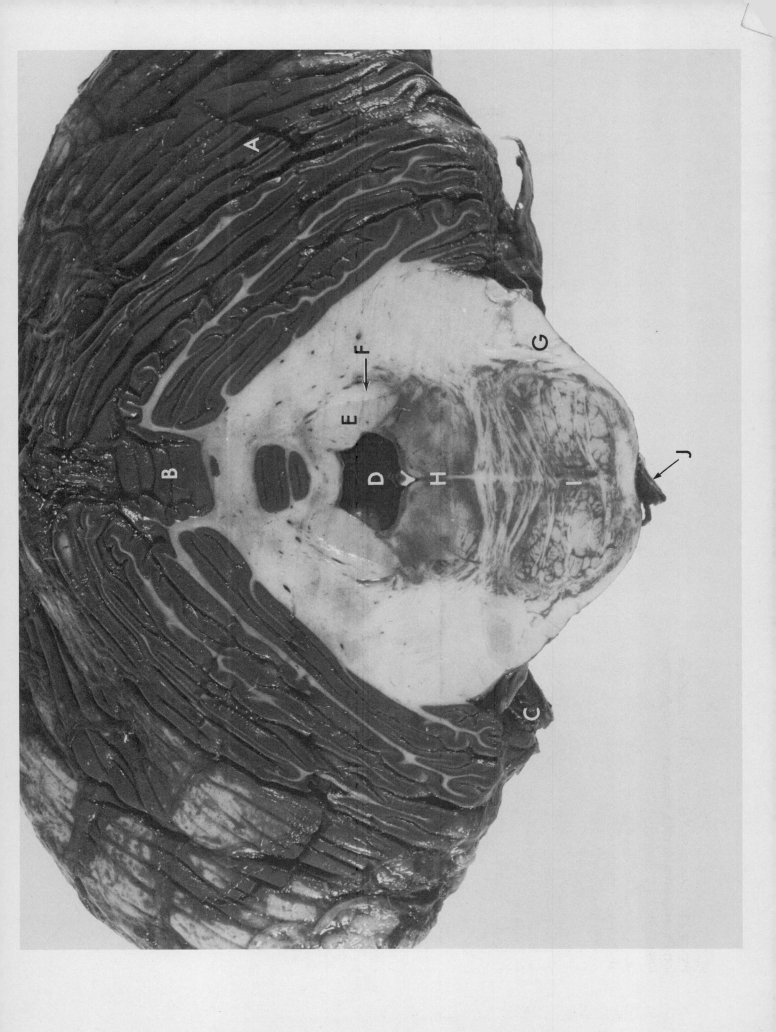

Figure 32. Transverse Section of the Medulla and Cerebellum Passing Through the Upper Portion of the Medulla Oblongata (×2)

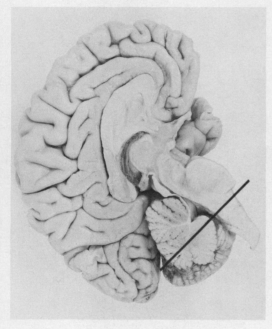

A. Cerebellar cortex (gray matter)
B. Medullary body (central white matter)
C. Cerebellar arbor vitae
D. Cerebellar folia (correspond to gyri of cerebrum)
E. Cerebellar fissures (correspond to sulci of cerebrum)
F. Dentate nucleus
G. Vermis
H. Fourth ventricle
I. Inferior olivary nucleus
J. Pyramidal tract (consists of corticospinal and corticonuclear fibers)

Can you locate:

Hypoglossal nucleus
Medial longitudinal fasciculus
Medial lemniscus
Inferior cerebellar peduncle
Inferior vestibular nucleus (and spinovestibular and vestibulospinal tracts)
Solitary tract and its nucleus
Spinal tract of trigeminal nerve (V)
Nucleus of spinal tract of V

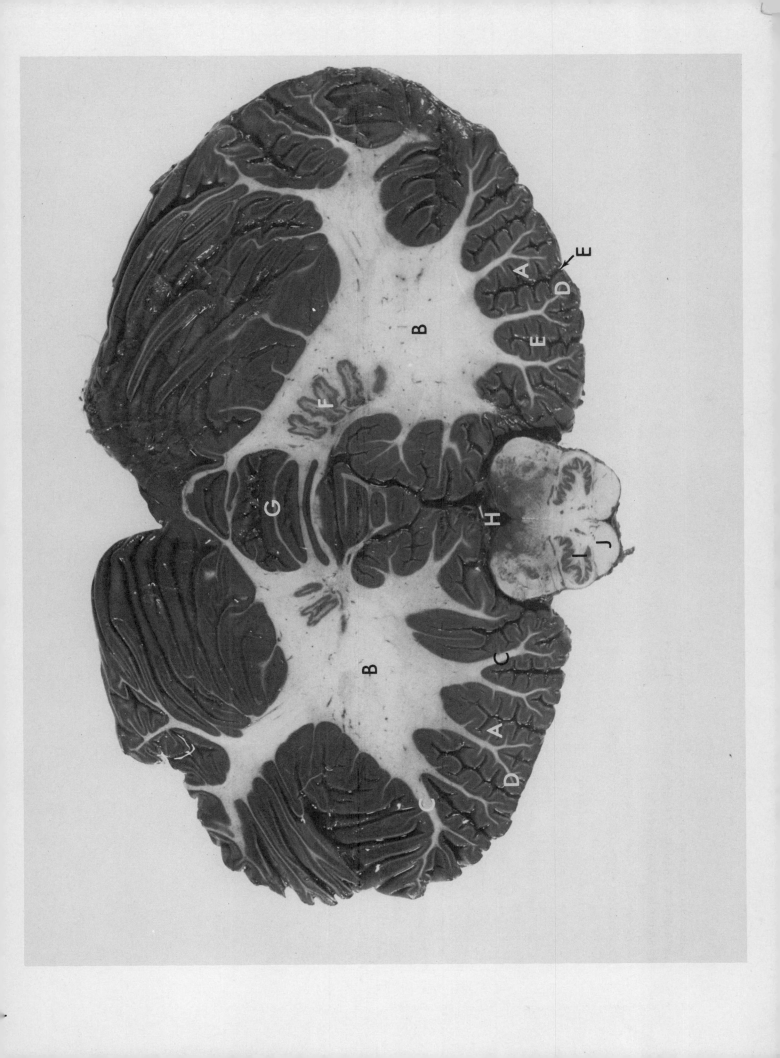

Figure 33. Transverse Section of the Medulla and Cerebellum Passing Through the Middle Portion of the Medulla Oblongata (×2)

A. Cerebellar cortex (gray matter)
B. Cerebellar arbor vitae
C. Cerebellar folia
D. Cerebellar fissures
E. Cerebellar hemisphere
F. Vermis
G. Pyramidal tract (consists of corticospinal and corticonuclear fibers)

Can you locate:

Nucleus and fasciculus gracilis
Nucleus and fasciculus cuneatus
Hypoglossal nucleus
Medial longitudinal fasciculus
Medial lemniscus
Spinal tract of trigeminal nerve (V)
Nucleus of spinal tract of V

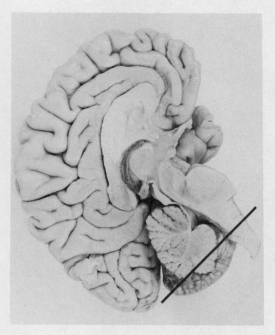

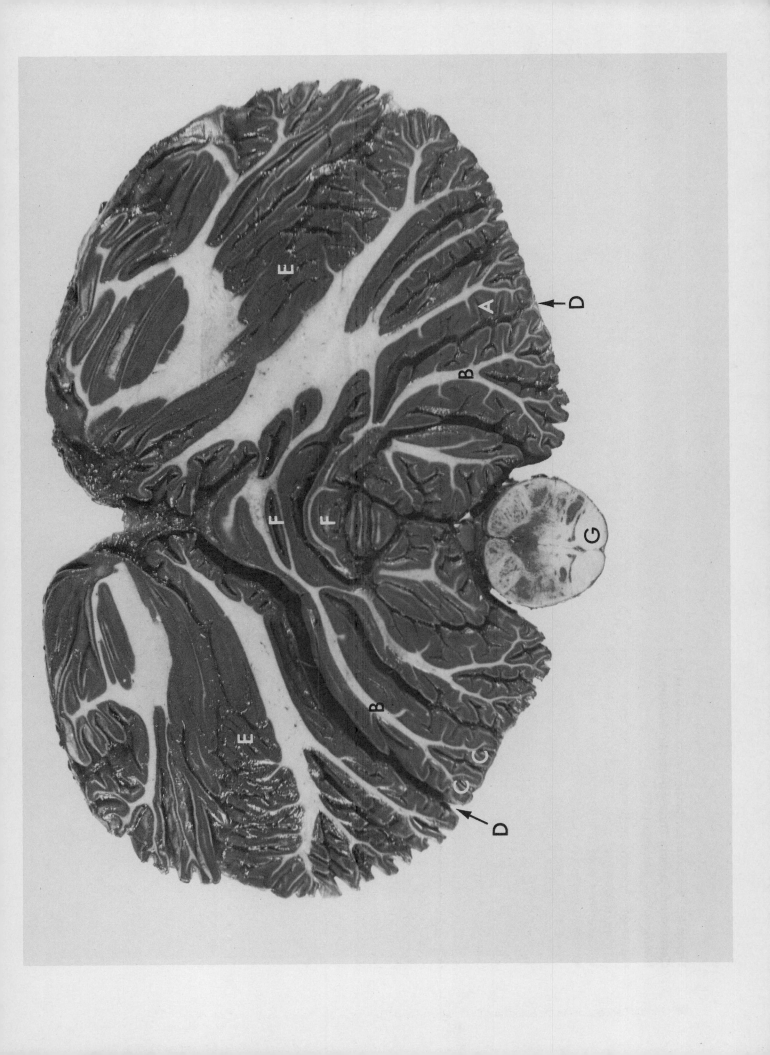

**TRANSVERSE SECTIONS OF THE SPINAL CORD
(Stained with a Modification of the Weil-Weigert Stain)**

Figure 34. Transverse Section of the Lowest Part (Conus Medullaris) of the Spinal Cord Passing Through the Coccygeal Region of the Cord and the Nerve Rootlets of the Cauda Equina (×25)

A. Coccygeal region of the spinal cord
B. Pia mater
C. Nerve rootlets of the cauda equina
D. Arachnoid

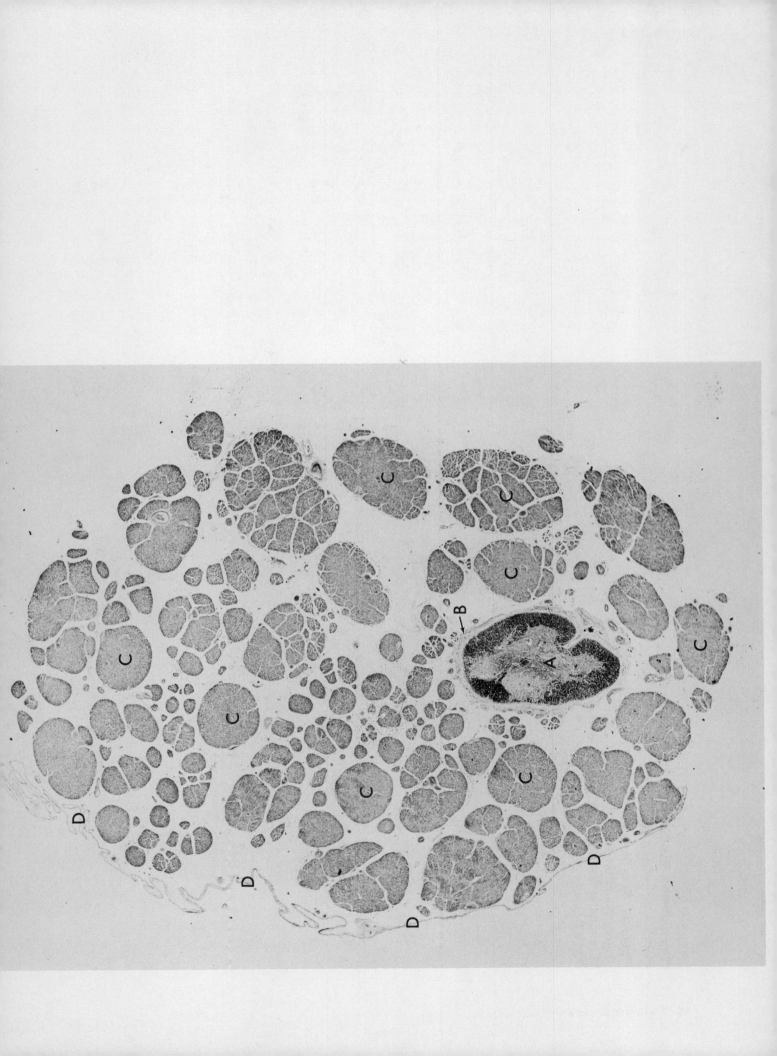

Figure 35. Transverse Section Through the Lower Sacral Region of the Spinal Cord (×20)

A. Anterior spinal artery
B. Anterior spinal vein
C. Posterior spinal artery
D. Posterior spinal vein
E. Posterior funiculus (fasciculus gracilis)
F. Lateral funiculus
G. Anterior funiculus
H. Anterior horn
I. Sacral parasympathetic nucleus (in intermediate column)
J. Posterior horn

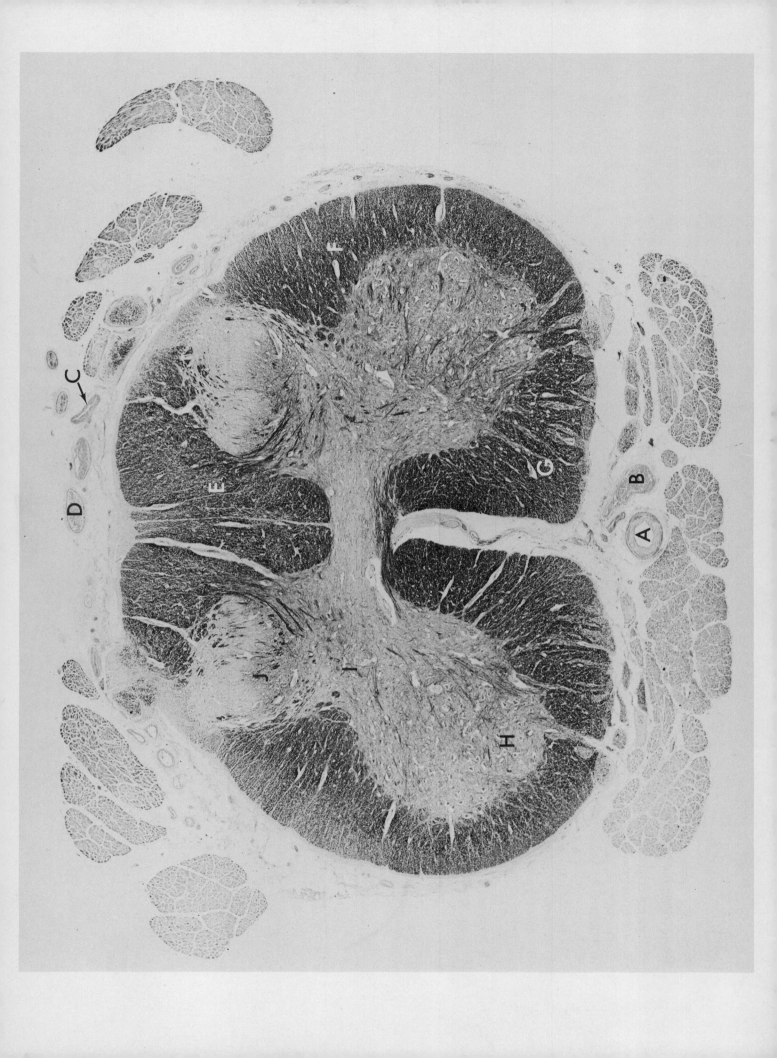

Figure 36. Transverse Section Through the Upper Sacral Region of the Spinal Cord (×20)

A. Dorsal root
B. Ventral root
C. Pia mater
D. Median sulcus
E. Median fissure
F. White commissure
G. Anterior funiculus
H. Anterior spinocerebellar tract
I. Lateral corticospinal (or pyramidal) tract
J. Fasciculus gracilis
K. Dorsolateral tract
L. Substantia gelatinosa
M. Posterior horn nuclei
N. Lateral division of anterior horn nuclei
O. Medial division of anterior horn nuclei

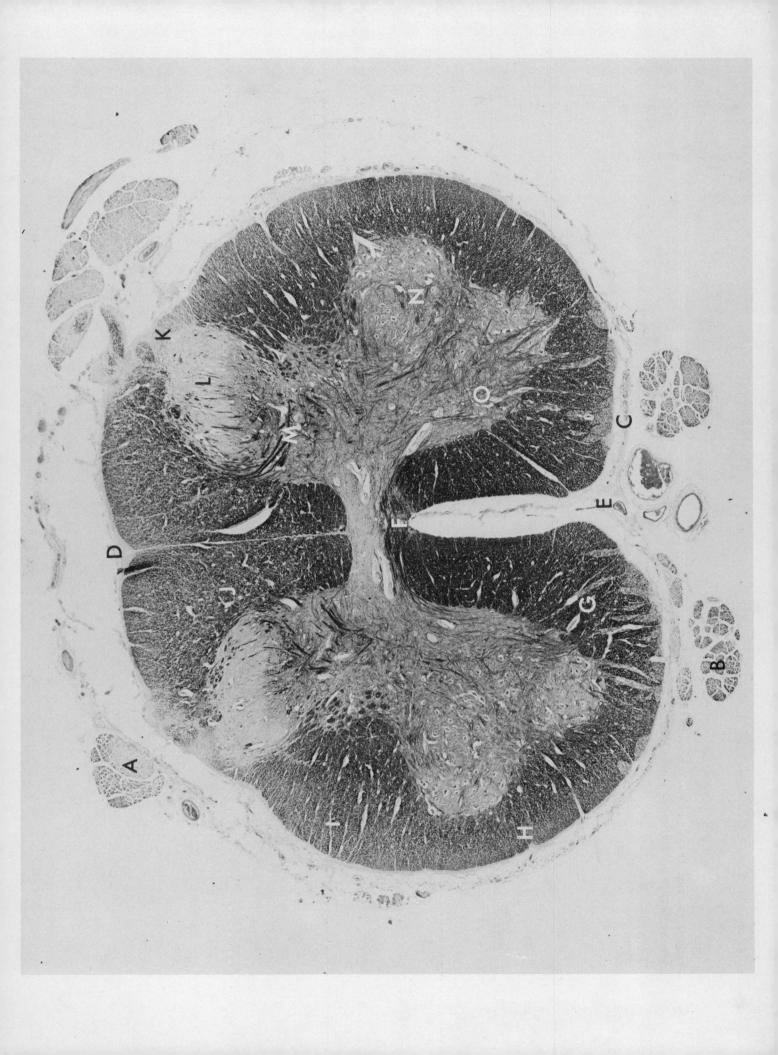

Figure 37. Transverse Section Through the Upper Lumbar Region of the Spinal Cord (×20)

A. Median sulcus
B. Posterior lateral sulcus
C. Median fissure
D. Anterior spinal artery
E. Anterior spinal vein
F. Anterior funiculus
G. Anterior spinocerebellar tract
H. Lateral spinothalamic tract
I. Lateral corticospinal (or pyramidal) tract
J. Fasciculus gracilis
K. Posterior horn
L. Thoracic nucleus
M. Intermediolateral and intermediomedial nuclei
N. Anterior horn

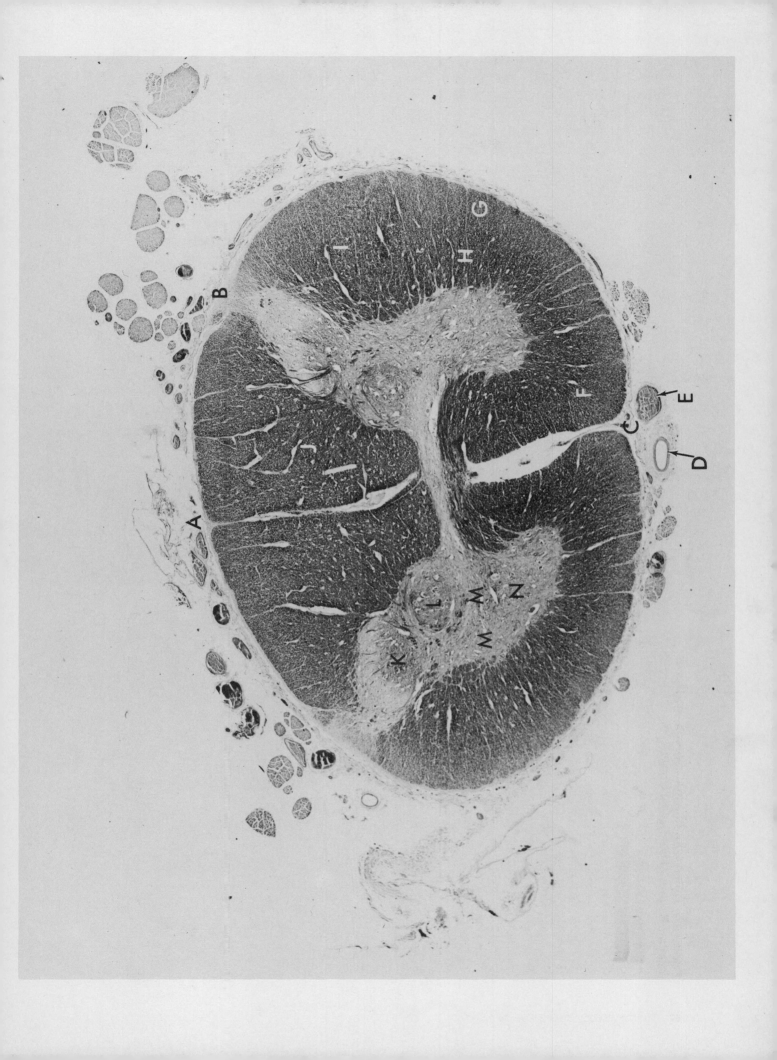

Figure 38. Transverse Section Through the Thoracic Region of the Spinal Cord (×20)

A. Fasciculus gracilis
B. Fasciculus cuneatus
C. Position of posterior spinocerebellar tract
D. Position of anterior spinocerebellar tract
E. Position of lateral corticospinal (or pyramidal) tract
F. Position of lateral spinothalamic tract
G. Position of vestibulospinal tract
H. Position of anterior spinothalamic tract
I. Position of anterior corticospinal (or pyramidal) tract
J. Posterior horn
K. Lateral horn
L. Anterior horn
M. Medial division of anterior horn nuclei
N. Intermediolateral nucleus of intermediate (gray) column
O. Intermediomedial nucleus of intermediate (gray) column
P. Thoracic nucleus (nucl. dorsalis, Clarke's nucl.)
Q. Central canal

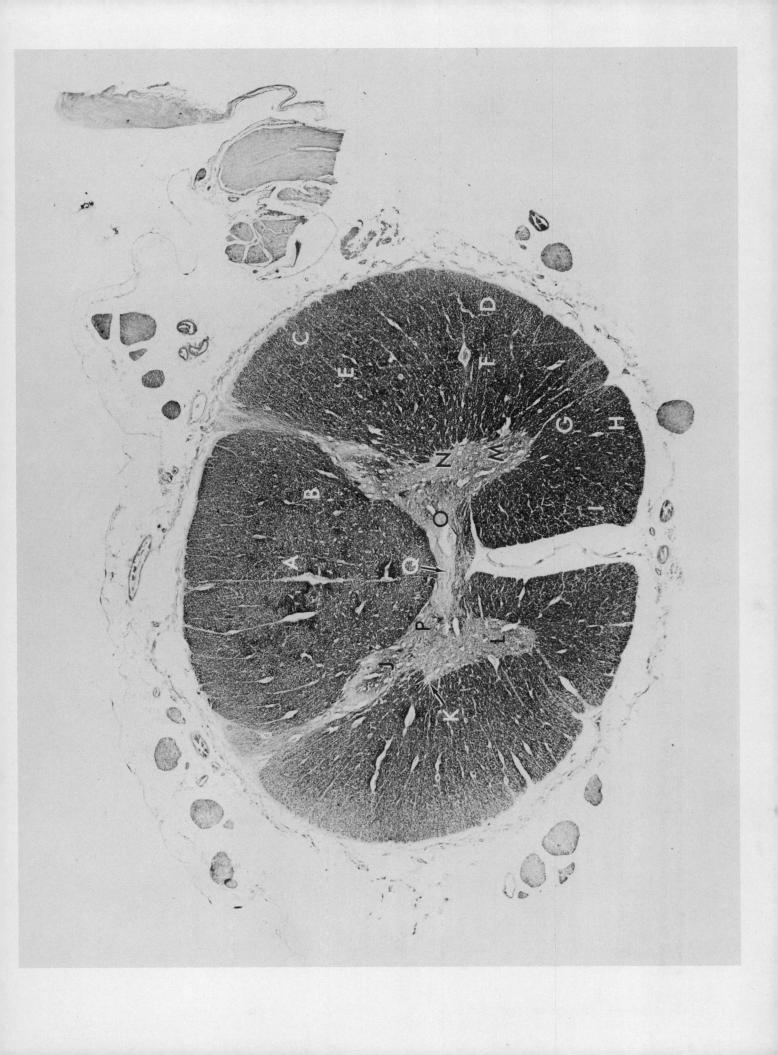

Figure 39. Transverse Section Through the Cervical Enlargement of the Spinal Cord (×18)

A. Dorsal root
B. Ventral root
C. Denticulate ligament
D. Median sulcus
E. Posterior intermediate sulcus
F. Posterior lateral sulcus
G. Median fissure
H. Posterior funiculus
I. Lateral funiculus
J. Anterior funiculus
K. Anterior horn
L. Posterior horn
M. Central canal
N. Fasciculus gracilis
O. Fasciculus cuneatus
P. Dorsolateral tract (Lissauer)
Q. Substantia gelatinosa
R. Posterior horn nuclei
S. Lateral division of anterior horn nuclei
T. Medial division of anterior horn nuclei

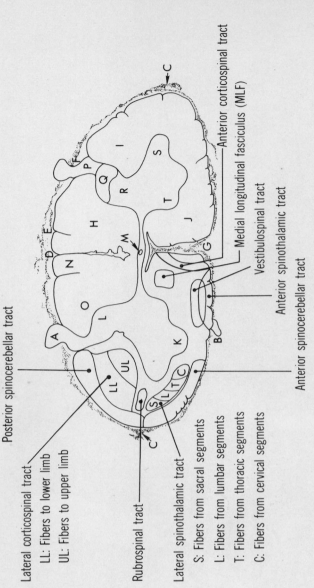

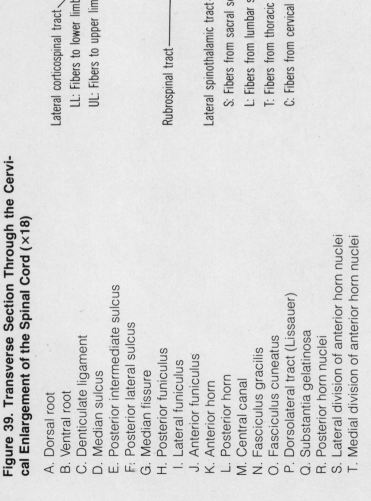

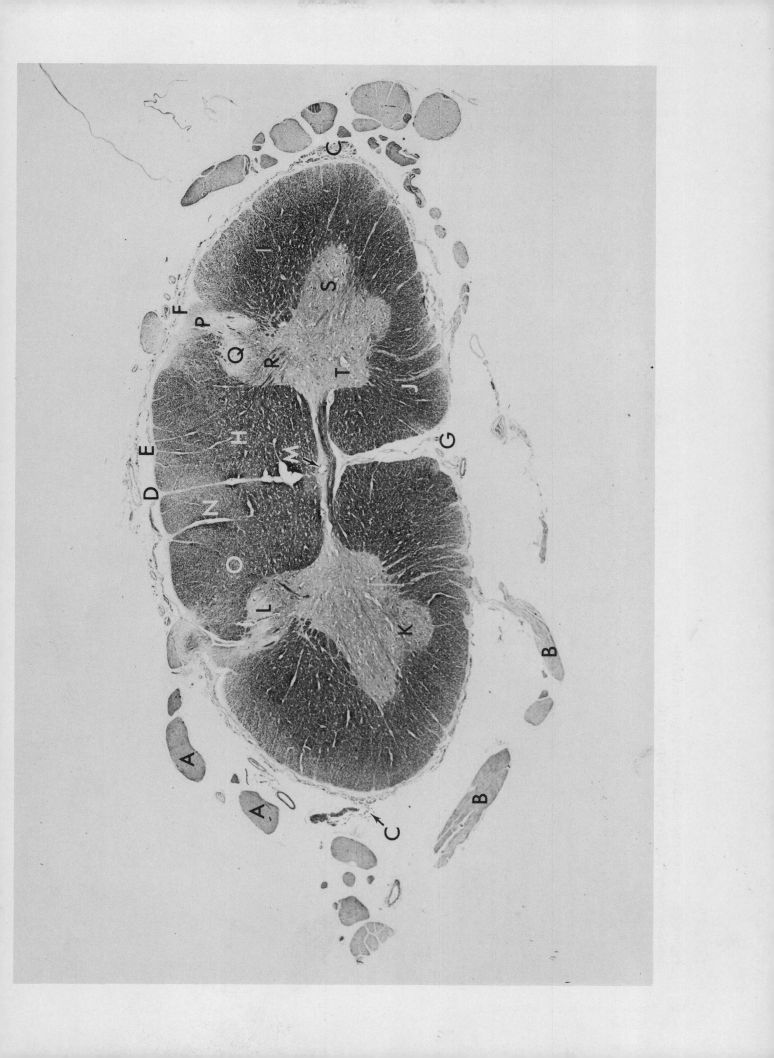

TRANSVERSE SECTIONS OF THE BRAINSTEM

Figure 40. Drawing of the Brainstem Indicating the Approximate Level and Plane of Figures 41–52 (Loyez Modification of the Weigert Stain)

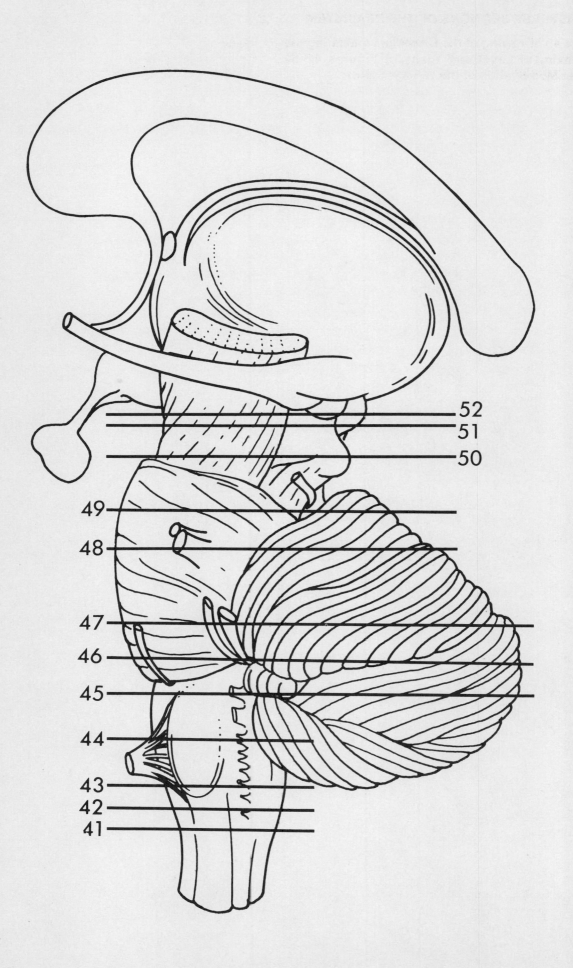

52
51
50

49

48

47

46

45

44

43
42
41

Figure 41. Transverse Section of the Transition from Medulla to Spinal Cord Passing Through the Decussation of the Pyramidal Tracts (×18)

A. Pia mater
B. Nucleus gracilis
C. Fasciculus gracilis
D. Fasciculus cuneatus
E. Spinal tract of trigeminal nerve (V)
F. Nucleus of spinal tract of V
G. Posterior spinocerebellar tract
H. Anterior spinocerebellar tract
I. Anterior horn of spinal cord
J. Medial longitudinal fasciculus
K. Anterior corticospinal (or pyramidal) tract
L. Pyramidal decussation
M. Lateral corticospinal (or pyramidal) tract
N. Central canal

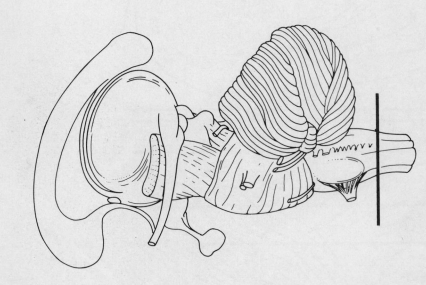

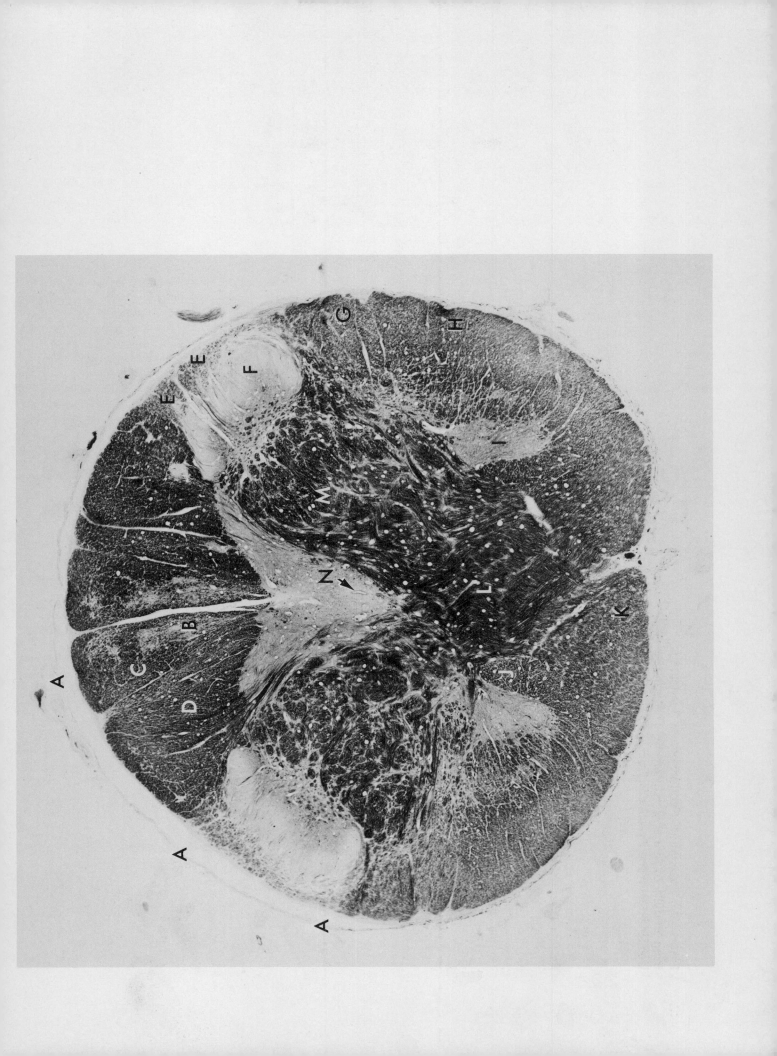

Figure 42. Transverse Section of the Lower Medulla at the Level of the Decussation of the Medial Lemniscus (×16)

A. Median sulcus
B. Fasciculus gracilis (from lower half of body)
C. Nucleus gracilis
D. Fasciculus cuneatus (from upper half of body)
E. Nucleus cuneatus
F. Spinal tract of trigeminal nerve (V)
G. Nucleus of spinal tract of V
H. Posterior spinocerebellar tract
I. Anterior spinocerebellar tract
J. Anterior and lateral spinothalamic tracts

K. Pyramidal tract
L. Reticular formation
M. Internal arcuate fibers
N. Medial lemniscus and its decussation
O. Solitary tract (*nucleus of solitary tract* is that part of the central gray substance surrounding the solitary tract)
P. Position of the dorsal (motor) nucleus of the vagus nerve (X)
Q. Hypoglossal nucleus
R. Median fissure

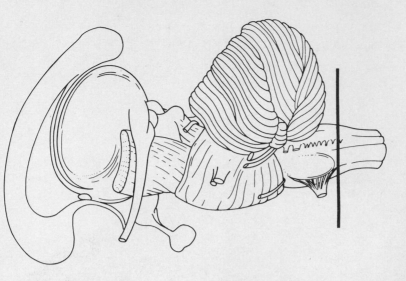

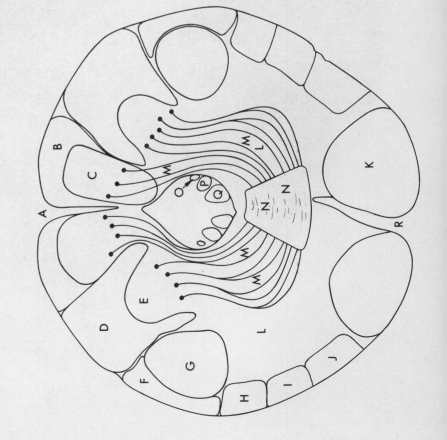

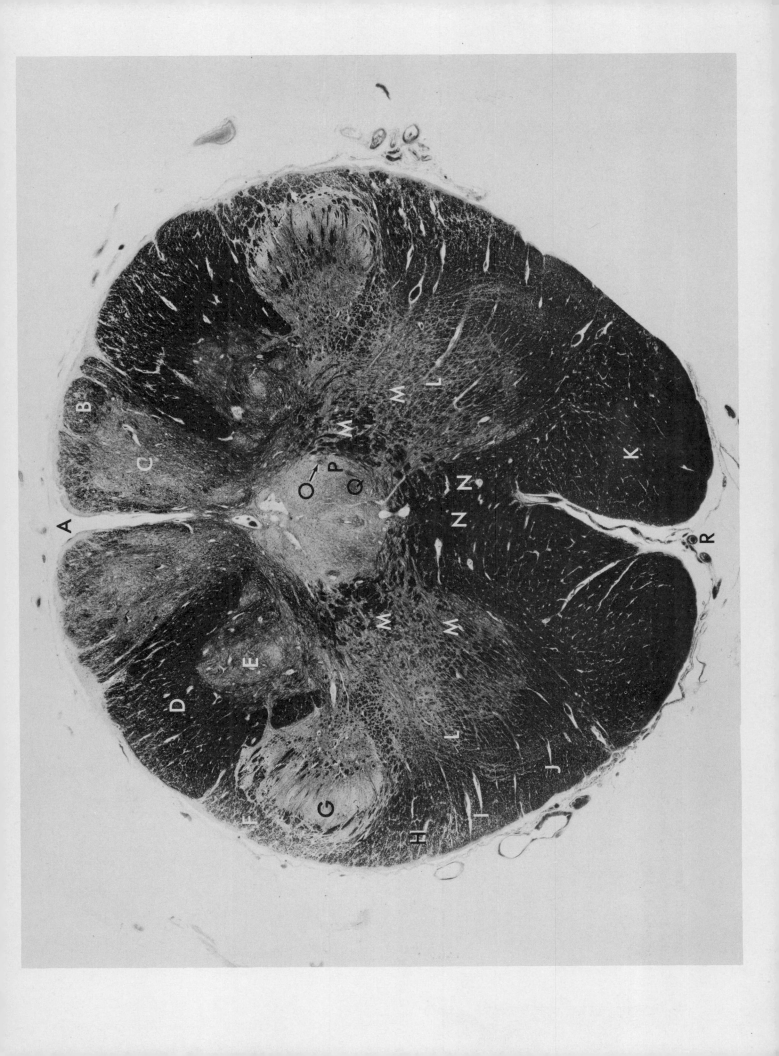

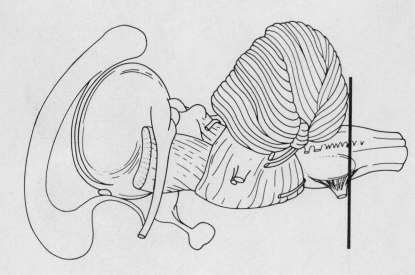

Figure 43. Transverse Section of the Medulla, Just Above the Obex, Passing Through the Lower Tip of the Olive (×12)

A. Fourth ventricle
B. Fasciculus and nucleus cuneatus
C. Posterior spinocerebellar tract
D. Anterior spinocerebellar tract
E. Anterior and lateral spinothalamic tracts
F. Inferior olivary nucleus
G. Pyramidal tract
H. Medial lemniscus
I. Hypoglossal nucleus
J. Dorsal longitudinal fasciculus
K. Dorsal (motor) nucleus of the vagus nerve (X)
L. Solitary tract (*nucleus of solitary tract* is the gray matter surrounding the tract)
M. Reticular formation
N. Medial longitudinal fasciculus (MLF)
O. Spinal tract of trigeminal nerve (V)
P. Nucleus of spinal tract of V

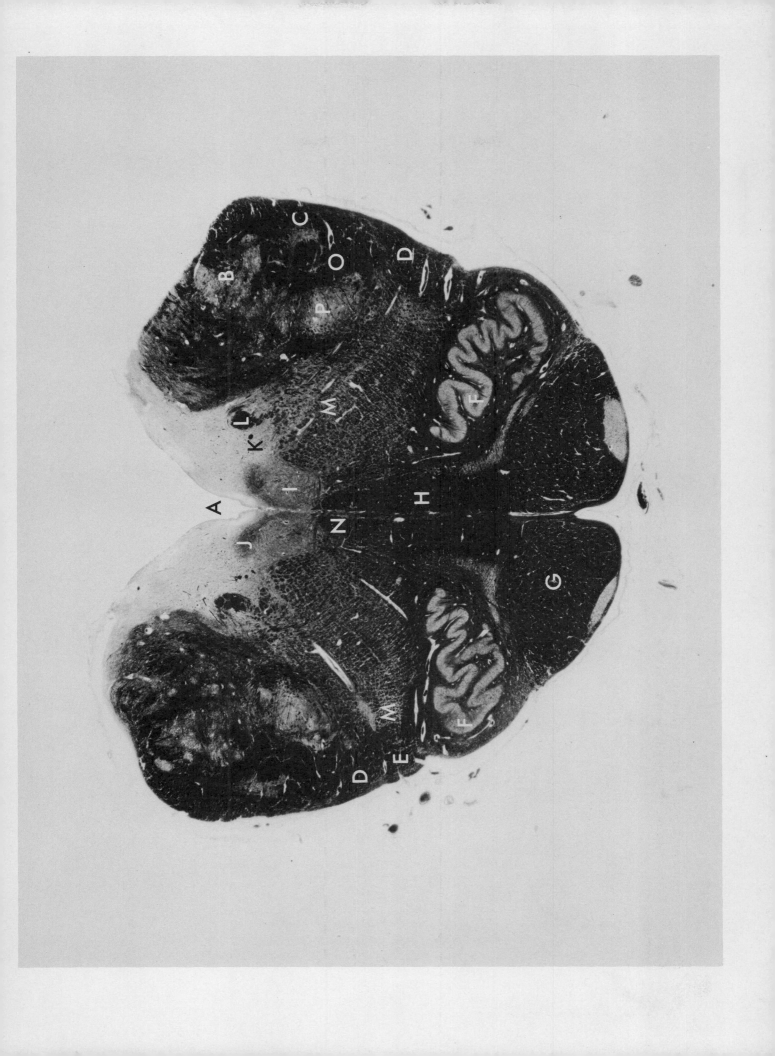

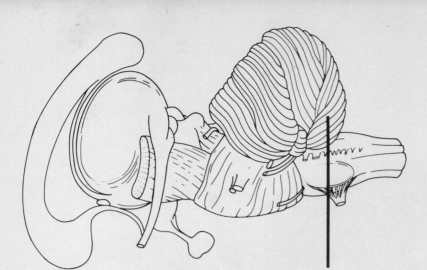

Figure 44. Transverse Section of the Medulla Passing Through the Middle of the Olive (×12)

A. Choroid plexus of fourth ventricle
B. Inferior medullary velum
C. Fourth ventricle
D. Pia mater
E. Inferior cerebellar peduncle
F. Spinal tract of trigeminal nerve (V)
G. Nucleus of spinal tract of V
H. Position of nucleus ambiguus
I. Anterior spinocerebellar tract and anterior and lateral spinothalamic tracts
J. Inferior olivary nucleus (forms the external bulge known as the *olive*)
K. Pyramidal tract (forms the external bulge known as the *pyramid*)
L. Medial lemniscus
M. Hypoglossal nucleus

N. Dorsal (motor) nucleus of the vagus nerve (X)
O. Solitary tract
P. Nucleus of the solitary tract
Q. Medial vestibular nucleus
R. Inferior vestibular nucleus (and spinovestibular and vestibulospinal tracts)
S. Accessory cuneate nucleus
T. Reticular formation
U. Medial longitudinal fasciculus (MLF)
V. Cuneate part of medial lemniscus (from upper half of body)
W. Gracile part of medial lemniscus (from lower half of body)
X. Fibers of hypoglossal nerve (XII)
Y. Fibers of vagus nerve (X)
Z. Position of fibers in the pyramidal tract to the face (F), upper limb (U), trunk (T), and lower limb (L)

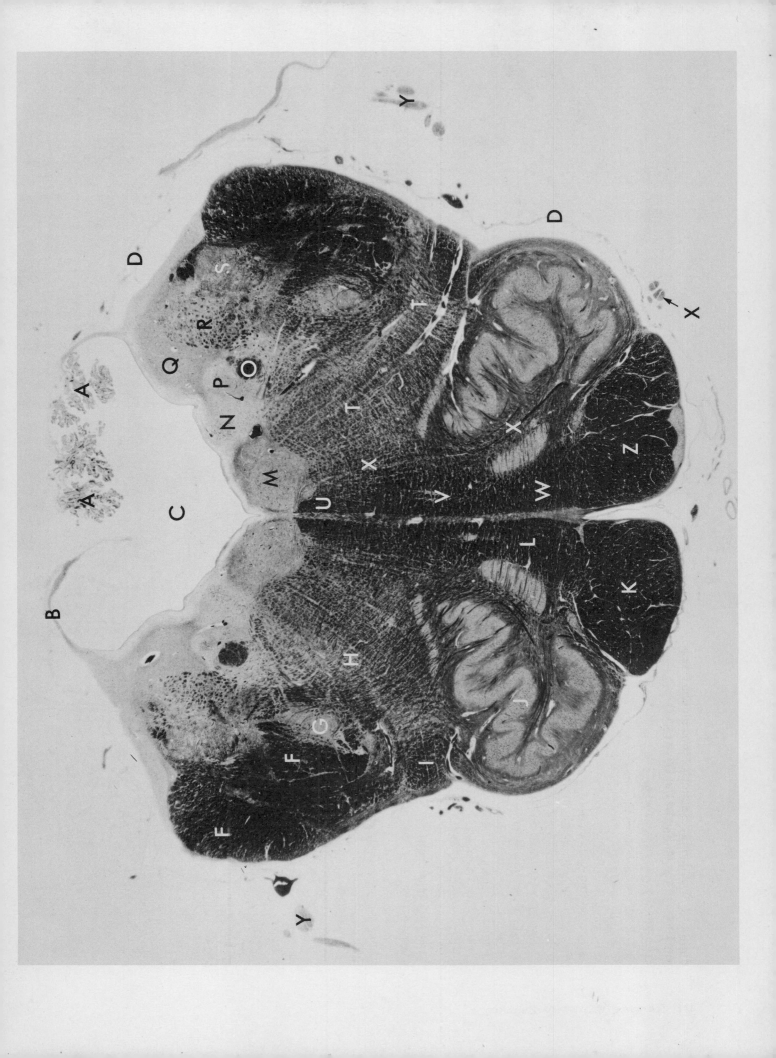

Figure 45. Transverse Section of the Upper Medulla, Near Its Junction with the Pons, Passing Through the Top of the Olive (×8)

A. Choroid plexus of fourth ventricle
B. Fourth ventricle
C. Medial vestibular nucleus
D. Inferior vestibular nucleus (and spinovestibular and vestibulospinal tracts)
E. Inferior cerebellar peduncle
F. Dorsal cochlear nucleus
G. Ventral cochlear nucleus
H. Vestibulocochlear nerve (VIII), cochlear part
I. Glossopharyngeal nerve (IX)
J. Solitary tract and its nucleus
K. Choroid plexus in the *lateral recess of the fourth ventricle*
L. Inferior olivary nucleus
M. Pyramidal tract
N. Medial lemniscus
O. Medial longitudinal fasciculus (MLF)
P. Spinal tract of trigeminal nerve (V)
Q. Nucleus of spinal tract of V
R. Inferior cerebellar peduncle entering the cerebellum

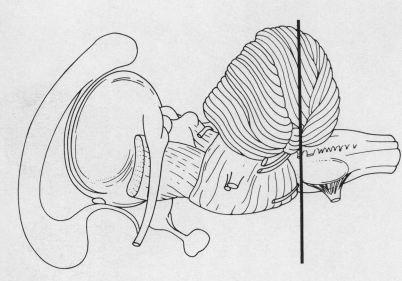

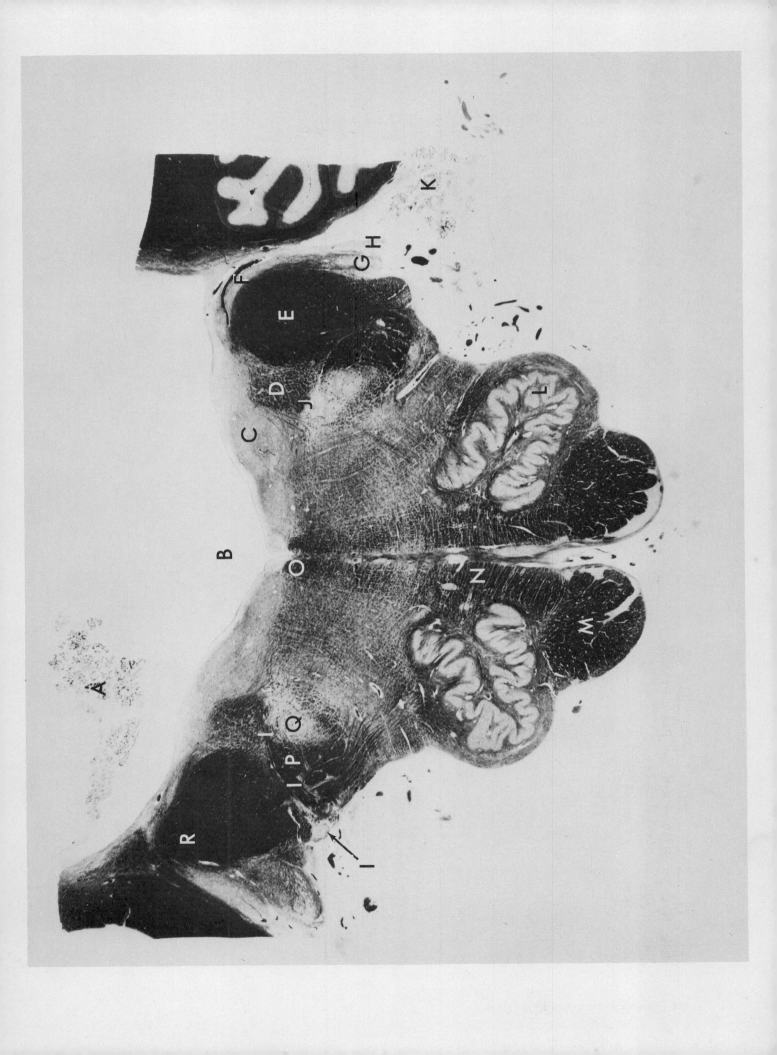

Figure 46. Transverse Section of the Lower Pons, Just Above Its Junction with the Medulla, Passing Through the Facial and the Vestibulocochlear Nerves (×7)

A. Nodulus of the cerebellar vermis
B. Dentate nucleus of the cerebellum
C. Fourth ventricle
D. Facial colliculus
E. Genu of facial nerve (VII)
F. Abducent nucleus
G. Lateral vestibular nucleus
H. Spinal tract of trigeminal nerve (V)
I. Nucleus of spinal tract of V
J. Facial nucleus
K. Lateral lemniscus
L. Superior olivary nucleus

M. Anterior and lateral spinothalamic tracts
N. Medial lemniscus
O. Central tegmental tract
P. Reticular formation
Q. Region of pontine center for horizontal gaze
R. Medial longitudinal fasciculus (MLF)
S. Pyramidal tract
T. Pontine nuclei
U. Middle cerebellar peduncle
V. Vestibulocochlear nerve (VIII)
W. Facial nerve (VII)
X. Fibers of the abducent nerve (VI)

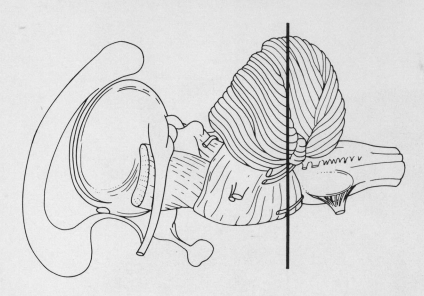

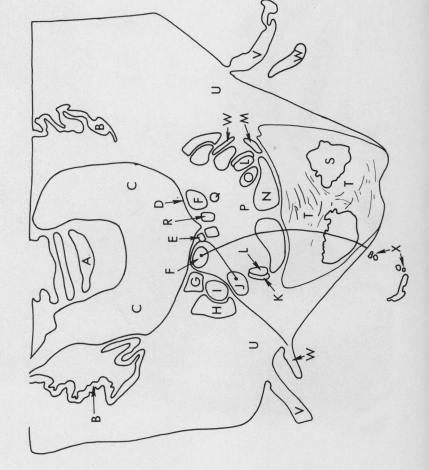

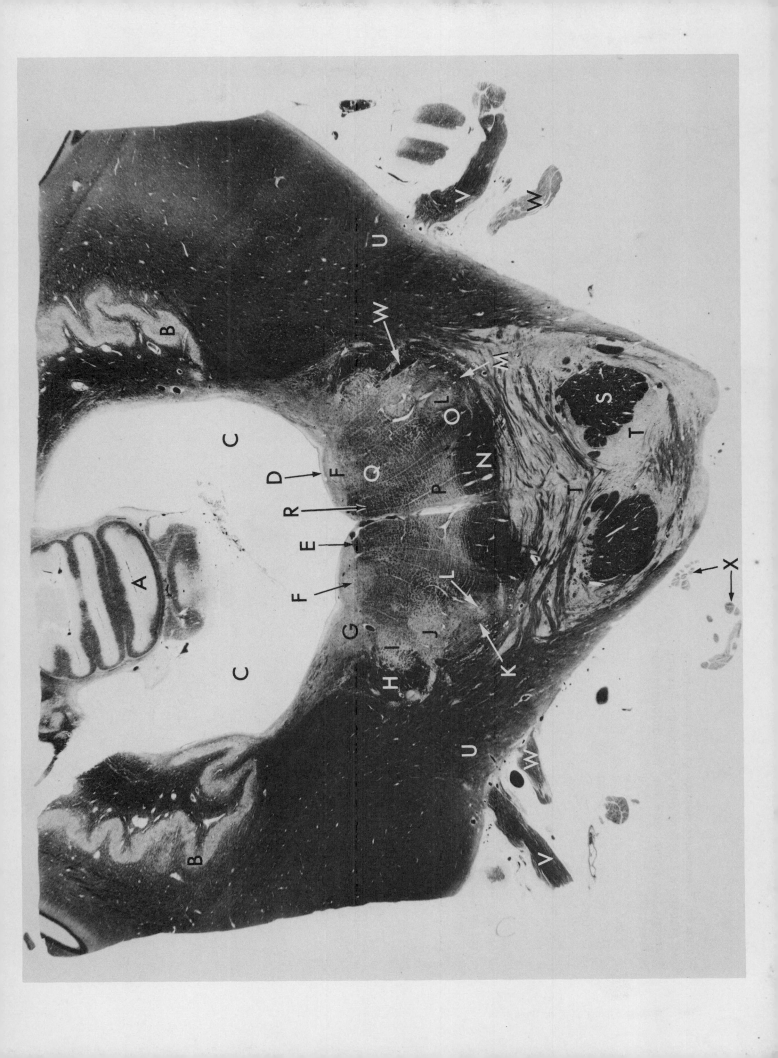

Figure 47. Transverse Section of the Lower Third of the Pons Showing the Intrinsic Nuclei of the Cerebellum (×6)

A. Fastigial nucleus of cerebellum
B. Emboliform nucleus of cerebellum
C. Dentate nucleus of cerebellum
D. Superior cerebellar peduncle
E. Fourth ventricle
F. Genu of facial nerve (VII)
G. Medial longitudinal fasciculus (MLF)
H. Superior vestibular nucleus
I. Spinal tract of trigeminal nerve (V) and its nucleus
J. Superior olivary nucleus (gray matter) and lateral lemniscus (white matter)
K. Anterior and lateral spinothalamic tracts
L. Medial lemniscus
M. Trapezoid body
N. Central tegmental tract
O. Reticular formation
P. Pyramidal tract
Q. Pontine nuclei
R. Middle cerebellar peduncle

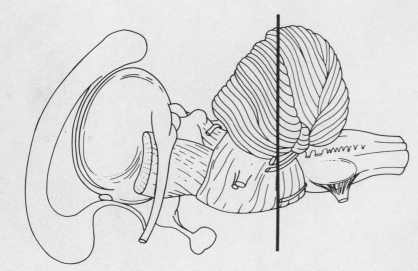

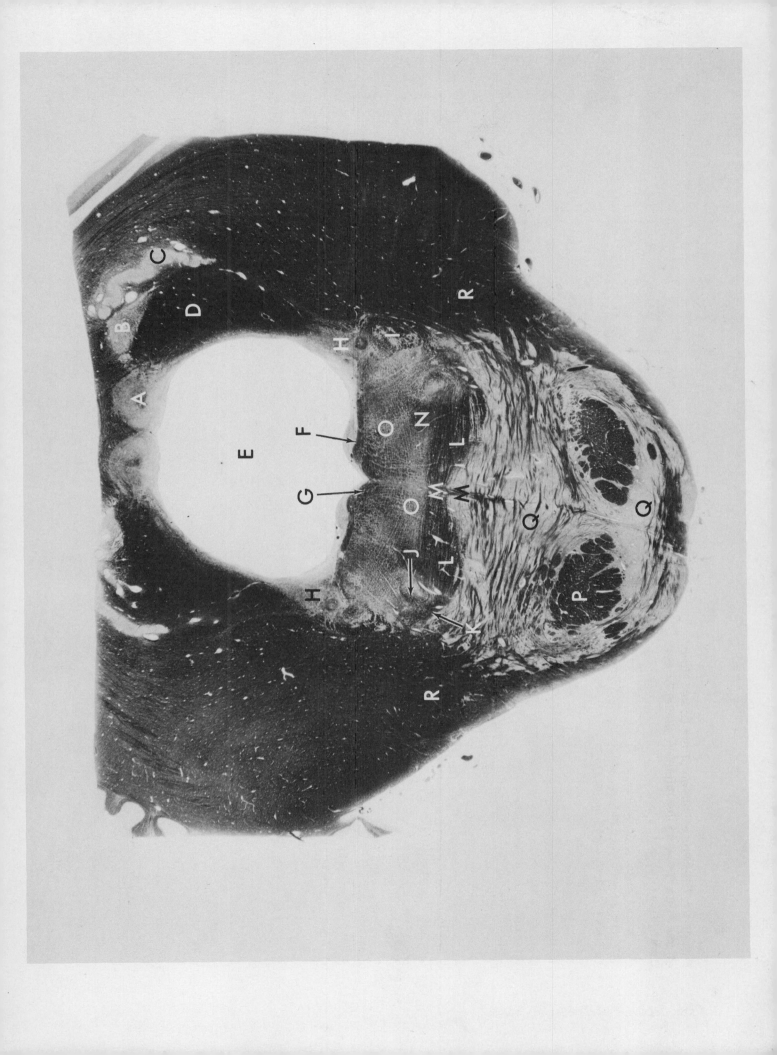

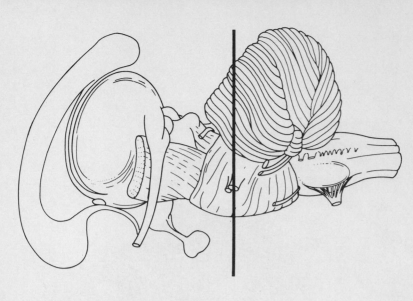

Figure 48. Transverse Section of the Middle Third of the Pons Passing Through the Trigeminal Nerve (×6)

A. Vermis of cerebellum
B. Hemisphere of cerebellum
C. Superior cerebellar peduncle
D. Fourth ventricle
E. Medial longitudinal fasciculus (MLF)
F. Motor nucleus of trigeminal nerve (V)
G. Principal sensory nucleus of trigeminal nerve (V)
H. Fibers of trigeminal nerve (V)
I. Central tegmental tract
J. Medial lemniscus
K. Secondary ascending gustatory tract (second-order taste neurons)
L. Cuneate part of medial lemniscus
M. Gracile part of medial lemniscus
N. Anterior and lateral spinothalamic tracts
O. Ventral trigeminal tract

P. Trapezoid body
Q. Reticular formation
R. Pyramidal tract and corticopontine fibers
S. Pontine nuclei
T. Middle cerebellar peduncle
U. Basilar artery (lying in the *basilar sulcus* of the pons)

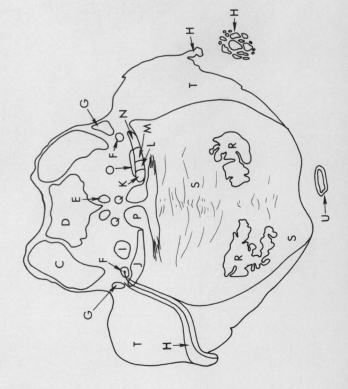

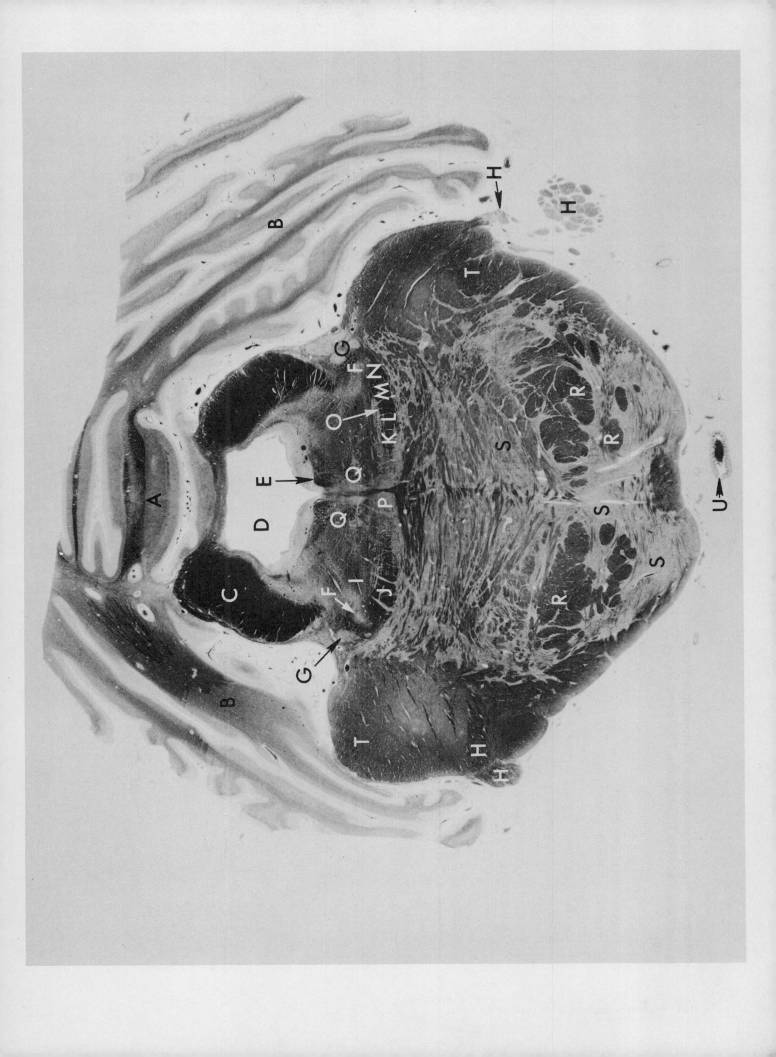

Figure 49. Transverse Section Through the Upper Third of the Pons (×8)

A. Superior medullary velum
B. Fourth ventricle
C. Mesencephalic tract of trigeminal nerve (V)
D. Nucleus of mesencephalic tract of V
E. Medial longitudinal fasciculus (MLF)
F. Central tegmental tract (the *dorsal trigeminal tract* is closely associated with this tract at this level)
G. Reticular formation
H. Superior cerebellar peduncle
I. Lateral lemniscus
J. Nucleus of lateral lemniscus
K. Anterior and lateral spinothalamic tracts
L. Gracile part of medial lemniscus
M. Cuneate part of medial lemniscus
N. Secondary ascending gustatory tract
O. Ventral trigeminal tract
P. Pyramidal tract and corticopontine fibers
Q. Pontine nuclei
R. Middle cerebellar peduncle

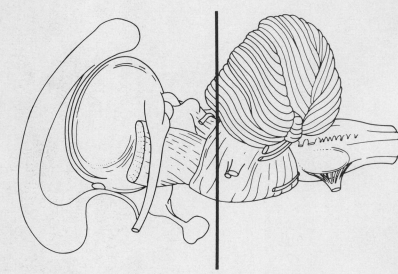

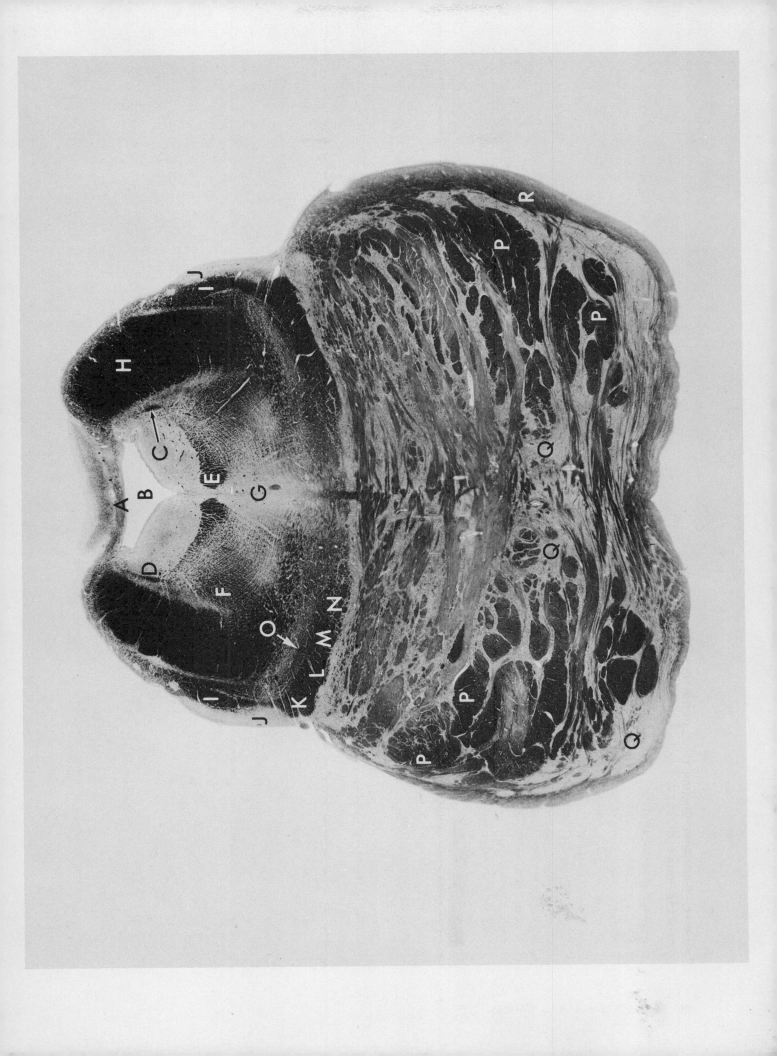

Figure 50. Transverse Section of the Midbrain Passing Through the Inferior Colliculus (×8)

A. Inferior colliculus
B. Lateral lemniscus (entering inferior colliculus)
C. Brachium of inferior colliculus (leaving inferior colliculus and projecting to medial geniculate body)
D. Lateral and anterior spinothalamic tracts
E. Gracile part of medial lemniscus
F. Cuneate part of medial lemniscus
G. Secondary ascending gustatory tract
H. Ventral trigeminal tract
I. Central tegmental tract (the *dorsal trigeminal tract* is closely associated with this tract at this level)
J. Reticular formation
K. Cerebral aqueduct
L. Central gray substance
M. Trochlear nucleus

N. Medial longitudinal fasciculus (MLF)
O. Decussation of superior cerebellar peduncles
P. Substantia nigra
Q. Crus cerebri
R. Frontopontine tract
S. Corticonuclear (corticobulbar) fibers of the pyramidal tract, eventually supplying muscles of the face, pharynx, larynx, tongue, etc.
T. Corticospinal fibers of the pyramidal tract supplying the upper limb
U. Corticospinal fibers of the pyramidal tract supplying the trunk
V. Corticospinal fibers of the pyramidal tract supplying the lower limb
W. Temporoparietooccipitopontine tract
X. Interpeduncular fossa

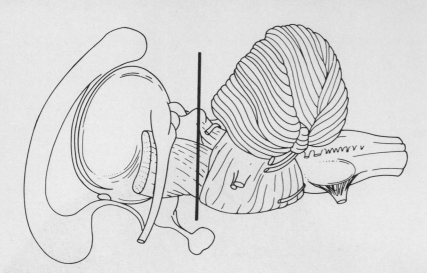

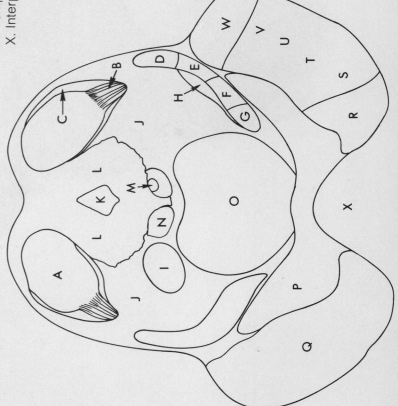

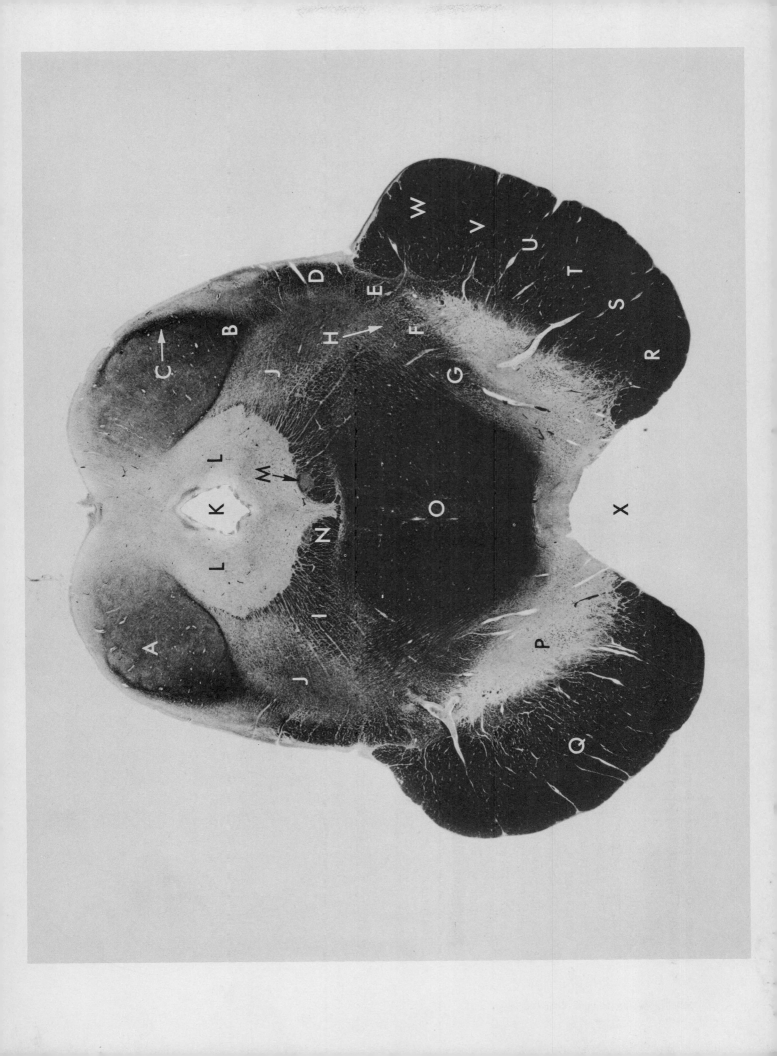

Figure 51. Transverse Section of the Midbrain Passing Through the Superior Colliculus and the Oculomotor Nerve (×8)

A. Superior colliculus
B. Brachium of inferior colliculus
C. Anterior and lateral spinothalamic tracts
D. Medial lemniscus and secondary ascending gustatory tract
E. Central tegmental tract and dorsal trigeminal tract
F. Superior cerebellar peduncle (above decussation)
G. Reticular formation
H. Cerebral aqueduct
I. Central gray substance
J. Position of accessory oculomotor nucleus (Edinger-Westphal)
K. Oculomotor nucleus
L. Medial longitudinal fasciculus (MLF)
M. Fibers of oculomotor nerves (III)
N. Substantia nigra
O. Crus cerebri
P. Interpeduncular fossa

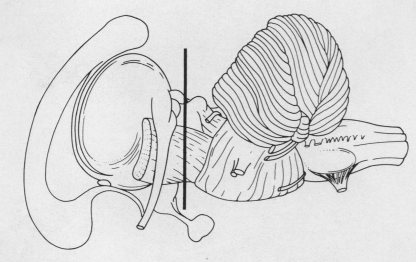

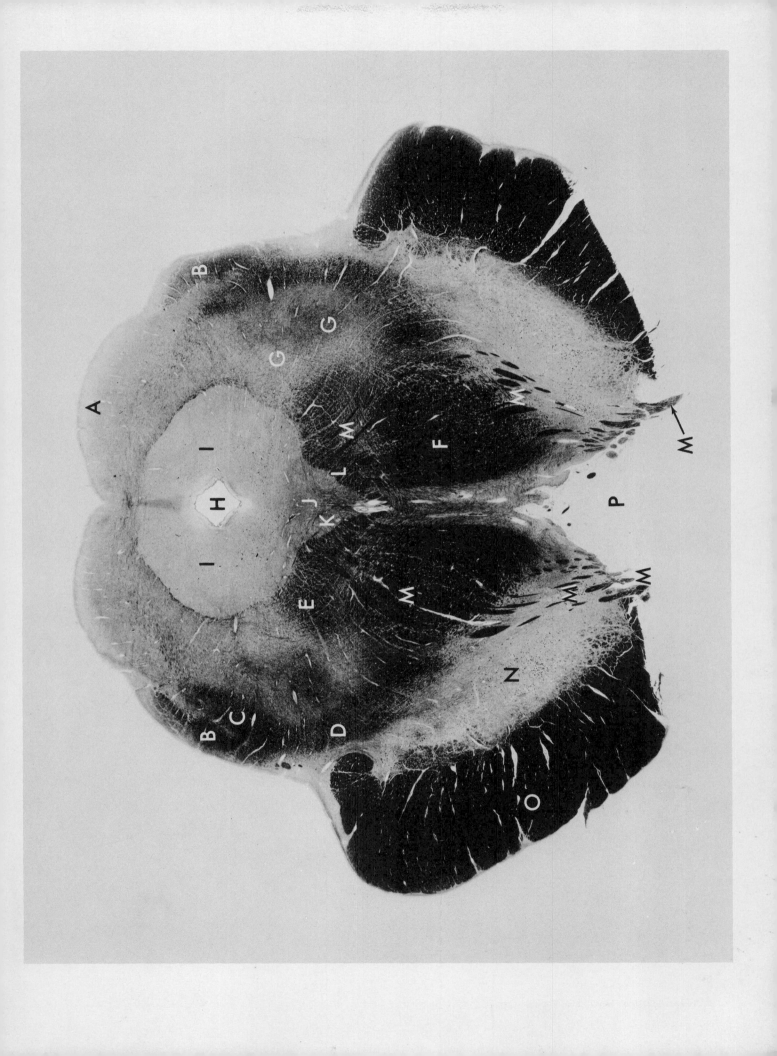

Figure 52. Transverse Section of the Midbrain Passing Through the Superior Colliculus (×8)

A. Superior colliculus
B. Brachium of inferior colliculus (entering medial geniculate body on the right)
C. Medial geniculate body of the thalamus
D. Reticular formation
E. Lateral and anterior spinothalamic tracts
F. Gracile part of medial lemniscus
G. Cuneate part of medial lemniscus
H. Secondary ascending gustatory tract
I. Ventral trigeminal tract
J. Central tegmental tract and dorsal trigeminal tract
K. Red nucleus
L. Habenulopeduncular tract (fasciculus retroflexus)
M. Dentatorubrothalamic tract
N. Cerebral aqueduct
O. Central gray substance
P. Position of accessory oculomotor nucleus (Edinger-Westphal)

Q. Oculomotor nucleus
R. Medial longitudinal fasciculus (MLF)
S. Fibers of oculomotor nerves (III) (difficult to see)
T. Substantia nigra
U. Frontopontine tract
V. Corticonuclear (corticobulbar) fibers of pyramidal tract to face and head and neck
W. Corticospinal fibers of pyramidal tract to upper limb
X. Corticospinal fibers of pyramidal tract to trunk and lower limb
Y. Temporoparietooccipitopontine tract
Z. Crus cerebri

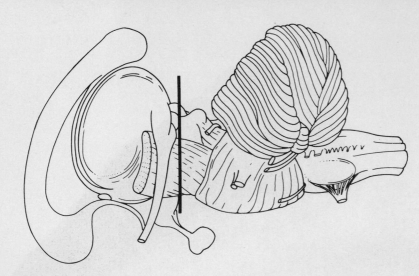

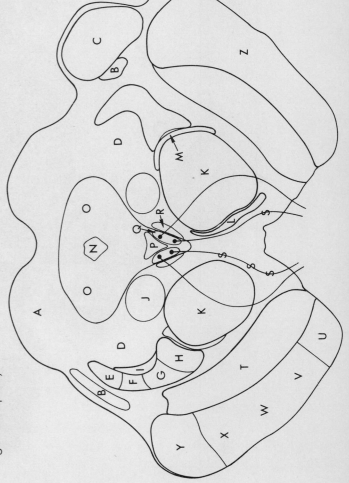

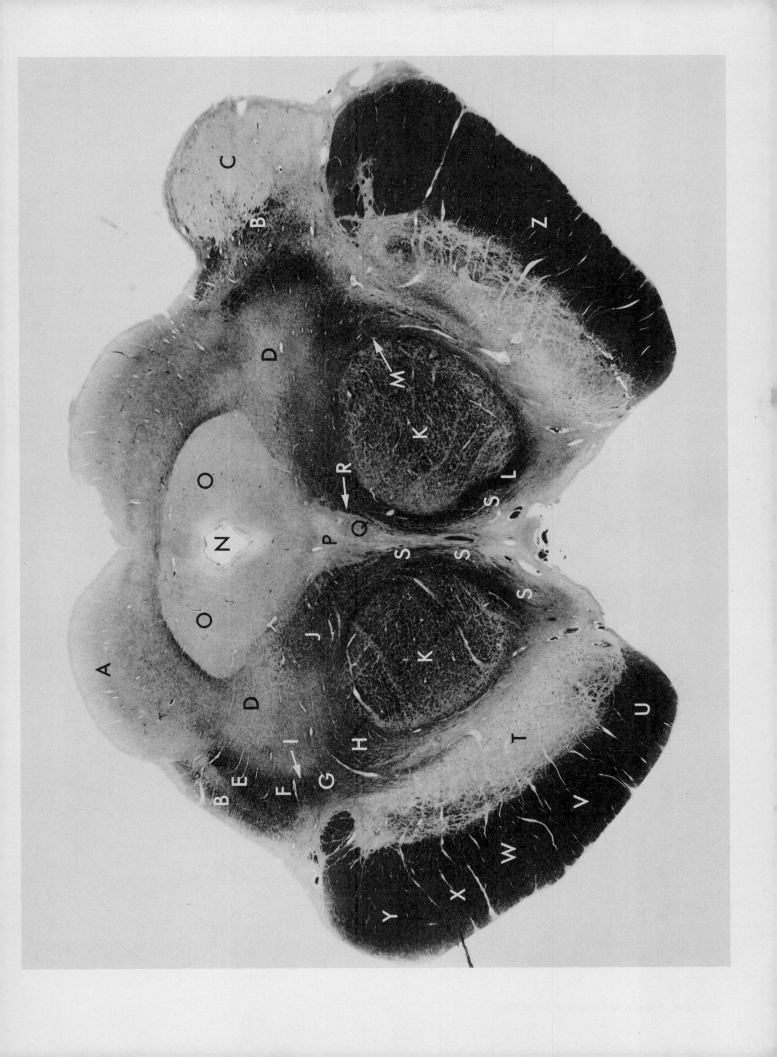

Selected References

Clark, R. G. *Manter and Gatz's Essentials of Clinical Neuroanatomy and Neurophysiology,* 5th ed. F. A. Davis Co., Philadelphia, 1975
A very nice, concise overview of the anatomy and physiology of the nervous system—some clinical correlations too. Recommended strongly for those interested in the nervous system.

Gardner, E. *Fundamentals of Neurology,* 6th ed. W. B. Saunders Co., Philadelphia, 1975
Another short, concise summary book (although not as short as Clark) on the nervous system. A little more detail than Clark.

Sidman, R. L., and M. Sidman. *Neuroanatomy: A Programmed Text,* Volume 1. Little, Brown and Co., Boston, 1965
This is a well-written programmed text and a very painless way to get into the nervous system. I recommend this book very strongly before a neuroanatomy course (either just before or just after reading Clark) or before you delve into the central nervous system in detail. Volume 2 is on its way.

Netter, F. H. *The CIBA Collection of Medical Illustrations,* Volume 1: *Nervous System.* CIBA Pharmaceutical Co., Summit, N.J., 1972
This book is a collection of 122 beautiful color illustrations of the nervous system (indeed, all the Netter-CIBA volumes are handsomely illustrated). Each illustration has a text describing what it's about. Clinical correlations too.

Chusid, J. G. *Correlative Neuroanatomy and Functional Neurology,* 16th ed. Lange Medical Publications, Los Altos, Calif., 1976
An intermediate-level, clinically oriented book on the nervous system. Pretty good.

Ranson, S. W., and S. L. Clark. *The Anatomy of the Nervous System,* 10th ed. W. B. Saunders Co., Philadelphia, 1959
This is an intermediate-level neuroanatomy book. Written for medical students.

Carpenter, M. B. *Human Neuroanatomy,* 7th ed. Williams & Wilkins Co., Baltimore, 1976
Similar but probably a bit better (and more detailed) than Ranson and Clark. A beautiful brainstem atlas is included at the back of the book. Recommended to those who are deeply interested in neuroanatomy.

Crosby, E. C., T. Humphrey, and E. W. Lauer. *Correlative Anatomy of the Nervous System.* Macmillan Co., New York, 1962
This is the Gray's Anatomy of neuroanatomy. It has almost everything you'll want to know about the central nervous system and a good deal you didn't know existed. I recommend this book if you intend to study the nervous system for the rest of your life, but not until you've been through some of the other books listed above (e.g., Clark, Sidman and Sidman, Carpenter). Many references included.

Curtis, B. A., S. Jacobson, and E. M. Marcus. *An Introduction to the Neurosciences.* W. B. Saunders Co., Philadelphia, 1972
This is an integrated text covering neurophysiology, neuropathology, and neurology as well as neuroanatomy. It has a series of excellent case studies scattered throughout the text.

Gay, A. J., N. M. Newman, J. L. Keltner, and M. H. Stroud. *Eye Movement Disorders.* C. V. Mosby Co., St. Louis, 1974
This is an excellent book covering many aspects of eye movement. In addition to chapters on the different eye movement systems and the functional pathways controlling them, it contains sections on clinical examination, nystagmus, the vestibular motor system, and specific eye movement disorders. Highly recommended.

Englander, R. N., M. G. Netsky, and L. S. Adelman. Location of human pyramidal tract in the internal capsule: Anatomic evidence. *Neurology* 25: 823–826, 1975

Shipps, F. C., J. T. Madeira, H. W. Huntington, and R. D. Wing. *Atlas of Brain Anatomy for EMI Scans.* Charles C Thomas Co., Springfield, Illinois, 1975

New, P. F. J., and W. R. Scott. *Computed Tomography of the Brain and Orbit (EMI Scanning).* Williams & Wilkins Co., Baltimore, 1975

INDEX

Index

Page numbers in boldface indicate illustrations